Risk Assessment and Management in Mental Health Nursing

Edited by
Phil Woods
PhD, RMN, RPN

and

Alyson M. Kettles
PhD, MSc, BSc, RMN, RGN, PGCEA, RNT,
Dip Crim, ILTM, FHEA, FRSM

WILEY-BLACKWELL

A John Wiley & Sons, Ltd., Publication

This edition first published 2009
© 2009 by Blackwell Publishing Ltd

Blackwell Publishing was acquired by John Wiley & Sons in February 2007. Blackwell's publishing programme has been merged with Wiley's global Scientific, Technical, and Medical business to form Wiley-Blackwell.

Registered office
John Wiley & Sons Ltd, The Atrium, Southern Gate, Chichester, West Sussex, PO19 8SQ, United Kingdom

Editorial offices
9600 Garsington Road, Oxford, OX4 2DQ, United Kingdom
2121 State Avenue, Ames, Iowa 50014-8300, USA

For details of our global editorial offices, for customer services and for information about how to apply for permission to reuse the copyright material in this book please see our website at www.wiley.com/wiley-blackwell.

The right of the author to be identified as the author of this work has been asserted in accordance with the Copyright, Designs and Patents Act 1988.

Wiley also publishes its books in a variety of electronic formats. Some content that appears in print may not be available in electronic books.

Designations used by companies to distinguish their products are often claimed as trademarks. All brand names and product names used in this book are trade names, service marks, trademarks or registered trademarks of their respective owners. The publisher is not associated with any product or vendor mentioned in this book. This publication is designed to provide accurate and authoritative information in regard to the subject matter covered. It is sold on the understanding that the publisher is not engaged in rendering professional services. If professional advice or other expert assistance is required, the services of a competent professional should be sought.

Library of Congress Cataloging-in-Publication Data

Woods, Phil, 1963–
Risk assessment and management in mental health nursing / Phil Woods and Alyson M. Kettles.
    p. ; cm.
  Includes bibliographical references and index.
  ISBN 978-1-4051-5286-0 (pbk. : alk. paper)   1. Psychiatric nursing–Risk assessment.   I. Kettles, Alyson, 1956–   II. Title.
  [DNLM: 1. Mental Disorders–nursing.   2. Psychiatric Nursing–methods.
3. Risk Assessment–methods.   4. Risk Management–methods. WY 160 W896r 2009]
  RC440.W578 2009
  616.89'0231–dc22

A catalogue record for this book is available from the British Library.

Set in 10/12.5pt Palatino by Graphicraft Limited, Hong Kong
Printed and bound in Malaysia by KHL Printing Co Sdn Bhd

1   2009

Contents

Foreword   v
Contributors   vii

1   Introduction   1
    Phil Woods and Alyson M. Kettles

2   Risk Assessment and Management   9
    John Cordall

3   The Theory of Risk   49
    Alyson M. Kettles and Phil Woods

4   Instrumentation   77
    Phil Woods and Alyson M. Kettles

5   Risk to Others   109
    Phil Woods

6   Risk to Self   143
    B. Lee Murray and Eve Upshall

7   Risk of Substance Misuse   199
    Lois Dugmore

8   Conclusions   243
    Alyson M. Kettles and Phil Woods

    Index   253

Foreword

Assessing and managing risk is a core part of the practice of all mental health nurses, regardless of whether they practice in a high-secure facility or in a primary care setting. It is certainly a truism that *'psychiatry is a risky business'*. This fact is continually emphasised in governmental publications and the colossal growth of research and professional papers on the subject of risk and mental health. Recent national reviews of mental health nursing in both England and Scotland have re-emphasised the importance of nurses' contribution to this activity. Psychiatry is innately risky because of the complexity of human motivation in the context of mental health problems and the resulting complexity of predicting future behaviour. This book provides a rigour to thinking about risk assessment and management, placing existing research findings in the context of day-to-day practice and, most importantly, ethical practice.

Mental health nursing has always been a profession that has had to balance the need to help protect people with mental illness, with the need to protect their rights to independence and self-determination. From the earliest times, nurses have been expected to successfully contain risk and have been held accountable when this has been unsuccessful. For example, in the nineteenth century nurses were fined if any of their charges managed to escape their care.

This book raises important issues regarding current perspectives on risk. In terms of proportionality, there are more forms of risk that nurses need to address than just those of direct risk from individuals to themselves through self-harm or harm to others through violence. This is an important point to be made, as the reality is that both suicide and homicide by people with mental illness are relatively rare events compared to the frequency with which individuals suffer abuse or neglect. Mental health nurses are open to pressures from the media and politicians to be over-reactive to perceived risk and consequently act in ways that are ultimately neither therapeutic nor in the long-term in the interests of people who receive mental health services.

Another significant point relates to attitudes to the management of risk, which have recently been the subject of much discussion. Mental health services are understandably concerned that they can be unfairly blamed when serious incidents such as suicides or homicides take place. Such unfair criticism can have the unfortunate effect of making healthcare services overly negative about the possibility of managing risk effectively in the majority of cases. The reality is that mental health nurses and others do effectively manage to work together with people with mental health problems to prevent harm. Every practicing nurse will be able to think of dozens of occasions when he or she has made an important contribution in this regard.

A key message within this book is that while statistical methods support the prediction of risk to a degree, it is through individual engagement and the consequent understanding of the unique motivations and thoughts of individuals that meaningful assessments are made and are the means through which much of the successful management of risk takes place. This book therefore valuably reiterates that mental health nurses need to combine the skills of rational evidence-based analysis with those of empathy for and sensitivity to the individual.

Neil Brimblecombe

Contributors

John Cordall RNMH, RMN, Cert. Research, MSc
John is a forensic nurse consultant at a medium-secure forensic unit in Yorkshire, England, and head of forensic nursing. His current clinical practice is focused on anger, risk and offence-related work, which includes leading and managing a cohort of clinical nurse specialists and incorporates strategic service development initiatives. He has previously completed the National Mental Health Nursing Leadership programme. He has presented papers nationally and abroad, and has written two previous nursing articles.

Lois Dugmore RMN, BA (Hons), MSc, MBA
Lois has been employed as a nurse consultant in Leicestershire for the last 4 years and previously worked for the Health Care Commission as an associate. She specialises in addictions and mental health and supports bringing the subject of substance use into mental health settings. Lois has published papers and contributed chapters to a number of books on substance misuse. Lois sits on the committee of a number of national groups including regional and national forums for dual diagnosis. Lois has a keen interest in mainstreaming sexual abuse within mental health services and is currently involved in delivering the Department of Health's violence and sexual abuse training for healthcare professionals.

Alyson McGregor Kettles PhD, MSc (Health Psychology) (London), BSc (Nursing Studies) (Dundee), RMN, RGN, PGCEA (Surrey), RNT, Dip Crim, ILTM, FHEA, FRSM
Alyson is the Research and Development Officer (Mental Health) for NHS Grampian and is based at the Royal Cornhill Hospital in Aberdeen, Scotland. She is also Honorary Senior Lecturer for the Centre for Advanced Studies in Nursing at the University of Aberdeen where she co-ordinates and teaches on modules for post-graduate Master's degrees. Her personal portfolio of research has had a forensic focus for more than the last decade, as a result of being the Link Tutor with Broadmoor Hospital while a nurse

teacher at the Frances Harrison College of Nursing in Guildford, Surrey, and at the University of Surrey. She is a well-known author of mental health and forensic nursing articles and books. Her research interests include assessment and interventions, such as risk and observation.

B. Lee Murray RN, BSN, MN, PhD(c)
Lee is an Associate Professor at the College of Nursing, University of Saskatchewan, and a Clinical Nurse Specialist in adolescent mental health. Her clinical practice includes individual and family therapy in the area of adolescent suicide risk and sexual health education for children and adolescents with developmental disabilities. She received the Saskatchewan Registered Nurses Association (SRNA) award for clinical excellence and has presented papers both nationally and internationally. She is a well-known author in the area of suicide risk. Her research interests include suicide risk assessment, sexual health promotion for adolescents with developmental disabilities, and interprofessional practice.

Eve Upshall BA (Psych Honors), BScN, RN
Eve is a practising acute care nurse and a sexual health educator for adolescents with developmental disabilities. She has been involved in a number of research projects including sexual health promotion, the sexual abuse of children/youths with developmental disabilities, developmental disability and willingness to abort, and child recall with regard to testifying in court.

Phil Woods PhD, RMN, RPN
Phil is an Associate Professor at the College of Nursing, University of Saskatchewan. He has an extensive personal portfolio of forensic and mental health-related research. He is a well-known author of mental health and forensic nursing articles and books. His specific research interests are risk assessment and management, and violence prediction.

Chapter 1

Introduction

Phil Woods and Alyson M. Kettles

Whether or not we like it, risk assessment and management is part of daily life for us. Every day, whether as a health professional or as a father, mother, son, daughter, husband or wife, and so on, we will be undertaking assessments of risk and consequently putting interventions in place to somehow manage or reduce those risks. One only has to do a quick literature search on risk to receive thousands of results from this, confirming Hayes' (1992) claim that for many years it has been an important concept in health, behavioural and social sciences, legal communities and the risk epidemic in medical journals (Skolbekken 1995). Indeed:

> '. . . one of the most lively areas of theoretical debate in social and cultural theory in recent times is that addressing the phenomenon of risk and the role it plays in contemporary social life and subjectivities' (Lupton 1999, p.1).

It is a clear fact within current mental health practice that risk assessment is very central to practice (Woods 1996) and indeed it is a requirement by society that we protect those who would need it and those that society needs protecting from. Doyle and Duffy (2006), amongst others, state how assessing and managing risk is a key task for mental health clinicians. Bloom *et al.* (2005) stress that it is an inherent dimension of psychiatric practice and Lewis and Webster (2004) that it is one of the highest profile tasks of mental health professionals. Rose (1998) informs how *'the language of risk now prevails mental health in the UK'*. Professor Louis Appleby, in the foreword to a recent Department of Health (2007) document on *Best Practice in Managing Risk*, states that it is clear that *'safety is at the centre of all good healthcare'* (p.3).

- So what is this thing called risk assessment?
- How do we do it?
- How do we do it well?
- What do we measure?

- How do we know if we are measuring the right things?
- How do we know if we have done it well?
- When do we do it?
- For whom do we do it?

These are just some of the many questions that roll off the tongue in relation to risk assessment and management. Those reading this book could probably also think of many more questions that they need answered. Well, it is hoped that this book may answer some of these questions and perhaps some readers may have themselves. It cannot be expected to answer all questions for all mental health nurses, but it can help to pave the way for them to consider their own practices and hopefully look further for answers that they may need.

Kettles (2004) discusses how health professionals understand risk in a variety of ways, but generally in mental health care, risk means a range of potential adverse events. Indeed, McClelland (1995) highlighted that one of the main problems that nurses face in their approaches to risk assessment, and its management, is that it is affected to a large degree by who defines the risk and how it is defined. This in itself is problematic in so much as if we as mental health nurses do not agree what is or what is not risk then how can we provide continuity of care across a range of services, and of course good risk management?

In this book, risk assessment and management have been viewed in the widest sense, although Chapters 2 and 3 will consider this more. As a starting point, risk can be considered as the probability of harm to self or others or a serious unwanted event; risk assessment is the process of determining this probability; and risk management is the process or intervention through which identified risks are reduced or alleviated. So risk can be considered from all perspectives: from deterioration in mental health status to suicide or homicide.

As mental health nurses and members of society it has to be noted that day by day we assess and manage risks well. How do we know this? Well, in our daily lives we manage to drive to work, cross the road and eat healthy diets, to name but a few examples. All these have potential risks involved in them and need us to put in place management plans to reduce these risks. In our professional lives, for example, when caring for a number of suicidal patients, why is it that they do not all manage to end their lives? Clearly we have assessed and are managing the risks associated with this well. What we are really doing is positive risk taking, *'weighing up the potential benefits and harms of exercising one choice or another'* (Morgan 2004, p.18). But how often do we really consider how we have done this?

Over the past 20 years or so mental health practice has changed considerably and this has developed specific challenges for the mental health nurse's role in risk assessment and management. Policy changes have seen a growing emphasis on community care rather than institutional care, where in the latter it was far easier to assess and manage risk through the added control and place of the sanctuary they provided for those cared for in them. Inpatient beds are becoming scarcer and periods of stay in hospital tend to be much reduced. These issues mean that those finding themselves in hospital are likely to be higher risk and demand enhanced skills from the mental health nurses who care for them. Conversely this also means that those who do not get admitted are perhaps more likely to be more risky than in the past, demanding different skills from the mental health nurses working in the community, perhaps with larger caseloads resulting from these changes. With this drive for community care and the related crisis intervention and assertive outreach services that have developed, risk assessment and management has been taken to a new level of difficulty.

According to the Department of Health (2001, pp.11–13), crisis resolution/home treatment teams provide a service for adults with severe mental illness with an acute psychiatric crisis of such severity that, without the involvement of a crisis resolution/home treatment team, hospitalisation would be necessary. Current policy in the UK (and throughout the world) has developed around the notion that people experiencing mental illness should receive treatment in the least restrictive environment, thereby minimising disruption in their lives. Crisis resolution/home treatment can be provided in a range of settings and offers an alternative to inpatient care. These services have developed to intervene with all four phases to crisis resolution:

- assessment
- planning
- intervention; and
- resolution.

As any and all of these phases are complex in many cases, effective risk assessment and management is a crucial yet challenging component.

In the same document, the Department of Health (2001) lays out clear implementation guidelines for assertive outreach services for those who have difficulty in maintaining lasting and consenting contact with services. Often they have severe mental health problems with complex needs and have difficulty engaging with services and often require repeat admission to hospital. Assertive outreach has been shown to be an effective approach to the management of these people and clearly good risk assessment and management is a crucial component of these services.

More recently, in the publication *From Values to Action: The Chief Nursing Officer's Review of Mental Health Nursing* (Department of Health 2006), key recommendation 10 (in relation to improving outcomes for service users) clearly states:

> *'Mental Health Nurses need to be well trained in risk assessment and management. They should work closely with service users and others to develop realistic individual care plans'* (p.5).

Throughout this key document many of the other recommendations are underpinned by issues of good risk assessment and management.

Similarly, the document *Rights, Relationships and Recovery: The Report of the National Review of Mental Health Nursing in Scotland* (Scottish Executive 2006) highlights one of the visions of mental health services as:

> *'Enabling, person-centred recovery and strengths-based focus with a move towards positive management of individual risk'*

with a mental health nursing response of

> *'Adopting frameworks for practice that promote values-based practice, maximising therapeutic contact time and the therapeutic management of individual risk'* (p.11).

Again throughout this key document many of the other practice and care issues discussed are done so in relation to good risk assessment and management. A clear stark message is therefore being sent by two major reviews of mental health nursing that risk assessment and management is high on the professional agenda.

As well as these developments in policy we can also observe that the provision of forensic services has grown vastly and more and more mental health nurses are finding themselves working within these areas with no specific advanced skills to prepare them for the task. Within these services there is a heightened pressure on mental health nurses to provide formal assessments of risk and related management strategies in very stressful patient situations. Some have taken up this challenge, however, using a systemic approach, such as the 'New to Forensic Programme' in Scotland (http://www.forensicnetwork.scot.nhs.uk/newtoforensic.asp).

When things go wrong in mental health services, inquirers who are tasked to find answers to what occurred frequently report failings in risk assessment and management. Often these are the results of tragic consequences. The corollary of such incidents is often a shift in public and political opinion and greater expectations placed upon nurses and other healthcare professionals. A tendency towards a more litigious society also places similar pressures on nurses and other healthcare professionals to provide accurate assessments of risk, which are often unrealistic. The result can be that clinicians will err on the side of caution and consider someone to be a higher risk than he or she actually is.

It is hoped that readers will find this book useful for their practice and take some thoughts or resources from it that can be used to enhance their current practice.

Topics covered in this book

In Chapter 2, John Cordall introduces some of the major discussion around risk assessment and management in mental health nursing. He sets forth some interesting discussion, critical debate and crucial challenges for mental health nursing. Such topics are expanded in later chapters as:

- Why assess risk?
- What constitutes effective assessment?
- The need for training.
- Mental health nursing roles.

Alyson Kettles and Phil Woods, in Chapter 3, introduce some of the theory of risk. The focus is on the wider theoretical aspects of risk assessment and management. The chapter outlines many common terminologies and defines terms clearly. This is important because much confusion surrounds the term 'risk assessment'. Concepts of variables and how they contribute to predicting outcome are discussed, introducing some of the latest thinking in the field. The chapter introduces the concept of risk management and its relationship to the risk assessment process. It is important that these theoretical foundations are laid so they can be related in the rest of the book.

In Chapter 4, Phil Woods and Alyson Kettles highlight and discuss some of the many instruments and processes that are available to assess and manage risk. The chapter includes an analysis of the requirements for the instruments cited and appropriate situations for their use. There is discussion on the inappropriate use of instruments, both in terms of incorrect interpretation and infringement of copyright, or other publisher require-ments, such as training. The chapter also focuses on the detailed research required to develop such instruments and how good risk management is based on sound risk assessment and can be informed by the use of such instruments and processes described.

Phil Woods, in Chapter 5, discusses the issue of risk to others. One particular theme that is examined in depth is evidence of links between violence and mental health. This chapter discusses some of the demographic and clinical variables that are associated with such risk and the importance of the nurse–patient relationship in the risk assessment and management process. Forensic issues are also discussed, as many of the offending issues that those working in this area have to deal with are related to risk to others.

Through Chapter 6, Lee Murray and Eve Upshall examine risk to self and some of the strategies for assessment and management. The most obvious and catastrophic aspect of risk to self is suicide, followed by varying degrees of self-harm (some of which are life threatening). Murray's approach to assessing and managing the risk of suicide and self-harm is a central component of the chapter. This approach, although developed in child and youth services, is equally applicable to adult services. Issues of self-neglect and vulnerability are also discussed. The chapter addresses such issues as diagnosis, developmental issues, gender, culture and the importance of the nurse–patient relationship in the risk assessment and management process.

In Chapter 7, Lois Dugmore discusses the risk of substance misuse. She unravels some of the complex issues surrounding the relationship between substance misuse and mental health. Policy issues are also identified. Early on in the chapter the effects of commonly abused drugs are discussed and the relative risk factors identified. The chapter contains a critical examination of the issues of assessment and management, care pathways, treatment options and harm reduction.

Chapter 8 is where Alyson Kettles and Phil Woods draw some conclusions, summarising the book and highlighting some key themes that it has contained. It is hoped this will help point readers towards other resources to develop their knowledge and understanding of risk assessment and management.

References

Bloom, H., Webster, C., Hucker, S. & De Freitas, K. (2005) The Canadian contribution to violence risk assessment: history and implications for current psychiatric practice. *Canadian Journal of Psychiatry*, **50**(1), 3–11.

Department of Health (2001) *Mental Health Policy Implementation Guide*. Department of Health, London.

Department of Health (2006) *From Values to Action: The Chief Nursing Officer's Review of Mental Health Nursing*. Department of Health, London.

Department of Health (2007) *Best Practice in Managing Risk: Principles and Evidence for Best Practice in the Assessment and Management of Risk to Self and Others in Mental Health Services*. Department of Health, London.

Doyle, M. & Duffy, D. (2006) Assessing and managing risk to self and others. In: *Forensic Mental Health Nursing: Interventions with People with*

'Personality Disorder' (National Forensic Nurses' Research & Development Group; eds P. Woods, A. Kettles, R. Byrt, *et al.*), pp. 135–150. Quay Books, London.

Hayes, M.V. (1992) On the epistemology of risk: language, logic and social science. *Social Sciences & Medicine*, **35**(4), 401–407.

Kettles, A.M. (2004) A concept analysis of forensic risk. *Journal of Psychiatric and Mental Health Nursing*, **11**, 484–493.

Lewis, A.H.O. & Webster, C.D. (2004) General instruments for risk assessment. *Current Opinions in Psychiatry*, **17**, 401–405.

Lupton, D. (1999). Introduction: risk and sociocultural theory. In: *Risk and Sociocultural Theory: New Directions and Perspectives* (ed. D. Lupton), pp. 1–12. Cambridge University Press, Cambridge.

McClelland, N. (1995) The assessment of dangerousness: a procedure for predicting potentially dangerous behaviour. *Psychiatric Care*, **2**, 17–19.

Morgan, S. (2004) Positive risk-taking: an idea whose time has come. *Health Care Risk Report*, October, 18–19.

Rose, N. (1998) Living dangerously: risk thinking and risk management in mental health care. *Mental Health Care*, **1**, 263–266.

Scottish Executive (2006) *Rights, Relationships and Recovery: The Report of the National Review of Mental Health Nursing in Scotland.* Scottish Executive, Edinburgh.

Skolbekken, J.A. (1995) The risk epidemic in medical journals. *Social Science and Medicine*, **40**(3), 291–305.

Woods, P. (1996) How nurses make assessments of patient dangerousness. *Mental Health Nursing*, **16**(4), 20–22.

Chapter 2

Risk Assessment and Management

John Cordall

Introduction

The concepts of risk assessment and management (which unless specifically noted will include risk taking) play a significant part in mental health nurses' (MHNs) everyday practice (Department of Health (DH) 2006), together with that of multidisciplinary teams (MDTs) (Jones and Plowman 2005), and will continue to do so, regardless of whether it is thought they should. This is informed by suggestion that specific risks in psychiatry are broad and incorporate:

- treatment effect adversity;
- self-harm;
- dangerousness to others; and
- risks to children

(Holloway 1998).

Despite this, there needs to be a balance between the needs of individual service users (and offenders) and the protection of the public (Prins 1999). A further consideration is that having a paucity of information and/or ignorance of such is tantamount to 'clinical gambling', with such gambles having the capacity to precipitate catastrophes (Snowden 1997).

The suggestion is not aimed at undermining the expanding amount of evidence-based research and practice within the professional press, but there does seem to be a paucity of information, from a mental health nursing perspective particularly (Crowe 2003). Focus is aimed at the need for improved consistency in the application of risk assessment and management techniques, given their centrality in mental health practice (Mason 1998; Kemshall 1999) and the pivotal role of MHNs in the interface between the two (Doyle and Dolan 2002).

However, here lies a dilemma. Despite the importance attributed to risk assessment and management, particularly in their protection of the welfare of mental health service users, that of the public, nurses themselves and the mental health services generally (Crowe 2003), perhaps a significant ring of truth is heard in the title *The 'Crystal Ball' of Risk Assessment*, one of Prins' (2005a) many eloquent works. Again, without being at all provocative to individuals contributing to the expansion of risk literature per se, yet acknowledging risk assessment and management's inexact nature as a science (Doyle and Dolan 2002), or even as an art rather than a science (Prins 2002), there seems to remain much debate about the concepts involved.

Admittedly, there have been developments since some of the late 1990s' proposals associated with factors such as (to name a few):

- what needs to be understood about risk assessment (Hollin 1997);
- the clarity of this and what should be assessed (Mason 1998);
- developing nursing risk strategies (Robinson and Collins 1999);
- proposals for a way forward (O'Rourke *et al.* 1997); and
- the lessons learnt from Inquiry reports (Reith 1998).

However, further work is needed. Perhaps, Grounds' (1995) suggestions that there are limits to professionals' risk knowledge, limits to their assessment of it, and imposed limits from service structure and ethos remain valid. Though he did reflect that progress may be made in the first two, it was not necessarily so with the latter, owing to drives towards community care and the security and public protection levels afforded when individuals are detained.

No doubt, significant reminders of previous criticisms of the mental health services for their risk failures (North East Thames and South East Thames Regional Health Authorities 1994; Petch 2001; Robinson *et al.* 2006) may be expected (though never condoned) by some in the mental health and criminal justice professions (Prins 2005b). However, reminders appear to be something that the public may neither want to hear nor think they should hear, given their expectations that professionals should get it right every time (Petch 2001). This is despite professionals themselves knowing that they cannot (Prins 2005b), and that risk assessments are not a talismanic charm against disasters (Maden 2003). There the dilemma remains and seems likely to remain for some time.

Standardising and simplifying risk language

Accepting the notion that the concept of risk can mean different things to different people (Doyle 2000; Kettles 2004), and MHNs, together with their

MDTs, are no exception, then having a consistent knowledge and understanding of the terms is important. This appears to be the case particularly in the context of assessing the risk of violence, if there remains truth in Webster *et al.*'s (2004, p.25) comment:

> *'At present there seems a regrettable tendency for researchers to talk one language and clinicians another. Researchers are often insensitive or unknowledgeable about clinical realities and clinicians too often are ill-informed about the results of dependable, informative research studies.'*

On a similar wavelength, Prins (2005b) proposed that a gradual change in language occurred well over 20 years ago, with the terms 'danger and dangerousness' being substituted by the notion of 'risk'. Regardless of the terminology used, individual professionals today are likely to recall where these terms have been used interchangeably, with a seeming innate understanding of what is (or in some instances is not) being referred to within the context of clinical discussions. However, does this simply add more misunderstanding to what seems, in this context, to be an already confused area of MHNs' professional practice?

Snowden (1997) suggests that 'risk' is a more attractive term than 'dangerousness', thus enabling objectivity and greater analytical robustness to focused questions aimed at identifying what the risks are, their severity and frequency, along with who may be at risk.

The Royal Society's (1992) use of risk terminology (cited in Prins 2005b, p.97) offers what could be interpreted as a useful framework for MHNs to work within, thereby achieving better consistency, and ultimately understanding, of respective risk issues.

- **Risk** – the probability of a particular adverse event occurring within a stated time period, or resulting from a particular hazard.
- **Risk assessment** – the study of decisions subject to uncertain circumstances, which was split into two components, risk estimation and risk evaluation.
- **Risk management** – decision making and implementation around risks, emerging from risk estimation and risk evaluation.

Without doubt, Prins (2005b, p.97) provides a most thought-provoking statement when he articulates the Royal Society's (1992) acknowledgement of the Health and Safety Executive's (1988) quote on 'tolerable risk':

> *'Tolerability does not mean "acceptability". It refers to the willingness to live with risk to secure certain benefits and in the confidence that it is being properly controlled. To tolerate a risk means that we do not regard it as negligible or*

something that we might ignore, but rather as something we need to keep under review and reduce still further if and as we can.'

The author feels that this epitomises what MHNs should use to improve clarity in their vital roles in respect of risk assessment and management, but just as important is for them to all use a similar language. This must also include an overt recognition of and wider broadcasting of evidence that validates their risk roles, but more importantly also openly informs the wider profession, their services and trusts and the public that working with service users' risks does have potential for things to go wrong. This may minimise some of the misperceptions about risks that were evident previously (Petch 2001), though it must be acknowledged that whether or not MHNs do this as well as they possibly can, it is likely that both risk assessment and management will continue to pose difficult questions, as highlighted by Mason (1998).

Why assess risks?

Based on the explicit statement by the United Kingdom Central Council for Nursing, Midwifery and Health Visiting (UKCC) (1998) to mental health and learning disability nurses, the risk management process is an integral part of their roles; it enables optimum care levels, values risk taking and attempts to reduce risks, though it is rarely possible to eliminate them. Clarity is contained in one UKCC paragraph!

Perhaps regarded by some (Grounds 1995; Cooke 2007) as a seminal work, Scott (1977) seems to have precipitated the continuing debate about what is now viewed as risk, with his proposals on the concept of dangerousness. Acknowledging that the discussion continues on the differences between dangerousness and risk per se (for example, Mason 1998; Prins 2005a), and that it should continue (though not in this chapter), one can draw a comparison with some of Scott's 30-year-old views on dangerousness and substitute the word 'risk':

'It (dangerousness) *is difficult to define, yet important decisions are based on it; . . . it is a term that raises anxiety and which is therefore peculiarly open to abuse, especially to over-response of a punitive, restrictive or dissociative nature. . . . The label, which is easy to attach but difficult to remove, may contribute to its own continuance. . . .'* (Scott 1977, p.127)

This could quite easily be affiliated to the premise of risk in today's professional world.

Duggan (1997) suggested that the assessment of dangerousness had been replaced by the assessment (and management) of risk, implying that the two are inextricably linked and inseparable, similar to the view of Kennedy (2001). The latter claimed that risk assessment is improvable on the basis that it informs appropriate risk management and ultimately mental health services overall, whilst Reed (1997) saw risk assessment not as a stand-alone initiative, but linked to a risk management plan, inclusive of review procedures.

Grounds (1995) had a much simpler perspective on clinical (risk) assessment, purporting it to be about making defensible decisions about dangerous behaviour, not primarily about prediction. West (2001), with regard to sex offender risk assessment, concluded that clinicians had little choice but to make decisions around dangerousness prediction and determining risk, given government, institute and public pressure.

However, risk assessment and management remains a central feature to meet service user needs and is thus a vital component in the Care Programme Approach (CPA) process (National Institute for Mental Health in England (NIMHE), 2004a) and, as such, falls into a healthcare trust's clinical governance arrangements (DH 1999a) as part of its continuous improvements in the quality and standards of care and treatment delivery.

The idea of formal risk assessment of people who have mental disorders is discussed in Taylor's (2001) *Expert Paper: Mental Illness and Serious Harm to Others*. In this (p.14), she highlights that an assessment process should include:

- risk of harm to others;
- risk to self;
- risk from others to patients (exploitation; for serious offenders – media exploitation and/or revenge attacks);
- risk of treatment non-compliance or absconsion;
- risk of substance misuse.

By contrast, Mason (1998) suggests that risk assessment in mental health practice has three main foci – violence risk, dangerousness and recidivism risk – though he perceived that there was a lack of concordance and strong confusion in the literature about what was being assessed and an interchanging of the terms' uses.

Comparatively, Lipsedge (2001) highlights that the greatest current concern for mental health services' risk management (and therefore risk assessment) is suicide and violence, but adds that most of the violence in communities is not committed by psychiatric patients, nor do those diagnosed with psychiatric conditions commit serious violent acts.

Kennedy (2001) proclaims that it is the mental health services' effectiveness as a risk management process for overall patient populations that really matters.

Importance is attributed to the many national drivers that have recommended the need to reduce and manage respective risks. These include:

- *Mental Health Policy Implementation Guide. Dual Diagnosis Good Practice Guide* (DH 2002a).
- *The National Suicide Prevention Strategy* (DH 2002b).
- *Mainstreaming Gender and Women's Mental Health* (DH 2003).
- *Mental Health Policy Implementation Guideline. Developing Positive Practice to Support the Safe and Therapeutic Management of Aggression and Violence in Mental Health In-patient Settings* (National Institute for Mental Health in England 2004a).

From a simple perspective, risk assessment may be aimed at achieving some balance in the responsibilities of service users, society, mental health services and healthcare professionals (Moore 1996), but at its heart must be the needs of service users, whether it be in terms of planning their future with them, maintaining their presence within their respective communities, projecting future treatment needs, or evaluating the necessity of continued detention for those who require it, amongst others. Regardless, Holloway (1998) acknowledges that the process requires attention to detail, which can be difficult within busy practice areas. However, he succinctly stresses this importance by proposing two clinically consistent themes emerging in Inquiry literature – failures in (1) understanding experiences and the social context of patients' inner worlds, along with (2) communicating associated information, particularly about dangerous behaviours, to key people. This sends out a powerful message, but should also act as a key factor in prompting and encouraging MDTs to improve their risk assessment and management skills through incorporating lessons learnt from such Inquiries (Reith 1998). Furthermore, when risk is not perceived as being managed, the likelihood of subsequent Inquiry is increased, with loss of trust in the healthcare professional to fulfil his or her role, making protest futile until improved risk management occurs (Maden 2005).

Contrastingly, Cooke (2007) claimed the following to be important in validated risk assessment:

- protection of the public;
- protection of staff and other patients/prisoners;
- equitable treatment of patients/prisoners;
- cost of holding individuals at too high a security level;
- targeting treatment resources where most needed.

Although these may have clarity and affinity for many, Bingley (1997) suggests that risk assessment also has accompanying moral and ethical challenges, together with potential costs for service users, their families, supporters and society. Regardless, he proposes that it must be afforded the highest priority, particularly for the competence of the assessment, along with subsequent management derived from its findings.

Szmukler (2003) seems to offer some support for Bingley's position in his discussion of the 'values' of risk assessment and management, together with their potential costs and benefits to society and particular social groups.

The idea of potential service user costs should not be underestimated. Robert (2006) offers personal experiences as a basis for highlighting the need for greater collaborative assessment and management of risk between MDTs and service users, which incorporates more empowerment, thus enabling potential negative conscious or unconscious influences, including stigma and fear of service users, to be minimised. Involving service users more, and thereby developing new systems of risk, will contribute to payoffs in public protection and service user care (Hollin 1997).

Crowe (2003) also alludes to some challenges in her thoughtful article on deconstructing mental health nursing risk assessment and management, concluding that the profession should examine its role in regard to those posing risks to others, thereby ensuring that practices correspond with responsibilities.

Although sad to say, and despite cognisance of the UKCC's (1998) position on defensible clinical practice, a further reason for risk assessment is seemingly the more commonplace questions regarding the availability, completion of and efficacy associated with risk assessments 'when things go wrong'. As if validating this, Prins (2005b) proposes that MDTs have to work within a blame culture, whereas Mullen (2002, p.296) makes an even starker statement:

> '*When tragedies occur, be they death or injury to the patient or inflicted by the patient, the question is now almost certain to be raised about whether adequate risk assessment procedures were in place to prevent, or minimise, such an untoward outcome. The question may be raised by administrators eager to place any blame that is going on the clinicians, by coroners seeking to apportion contribution to the death, by enquiries deciding who to pillory, and most egregious of all, by colleagues prepared to self-righteously point the finger of blame.*'

This is not to suggest that there should be a blame-free culture, as society itself is far from that (Alaszewski 1998), nor that the impact of a tragedy should be minimised (Reed 1997), but rather that we should strive for a just culture. This goes back to educating the public that professionals cannot get it right every time, as risk assessment remains a 'risky business'

(Prins 2002), prediction is not possible (Potts 1995) and risk assessments are fallible (Munro and Rumgay 2000). Yet, pro-rata, the thousands of risk decisions that are made in everyday mental health practice which go right are seemingly outweighed by those that go wrong. This is despite the *National Confidential Inquiry into Suicide and Homicide by People with Mental Illness* (DH 1999b) which highlights findings that within its sample of mental health service users who committed suicide, an individual's immediate risk of suicide was estimated as low or absent in 85% of cases at their last service contact. This is not to detract from the recognised failures the Inquiry articulated, but serves simply to flag up some of the hardships that professionals face. This needs to be uppermost in MDT thinking, along with the many other associated variables linked to practice. Perhaps Kemshall (1999, p.33) offers a balanced view of professionals' roles by claiming:

> *'Practitioners have an obligation to act responsibly and defensibly on risk, but not guarantee its prevention'.*

What constitutes effective risk assessment?

Is this an unanswerable question? If Petch (2001) is correct in proposing the stark reality that regardless of how good risk assessment tools are, either clinical or actuarial, professionals will not significantly impact on public safety unless mental health services generally improve, then yes, it is possibly an unanswerable question. Munro and Rumgay (2000) seem to offer a similar perspective, drawing on their examination of findings from public inquiries into homicides by people with mental illness. Their conclusion concludes that improved risk assessment has only a limited role in reducing homicides, with overall mental healthcare improvements suggestive as being the most effective preventative strategy therein.

Despite this initial discussion, the starting point for effective risk assessment and management has to be full service user and carer/family involvement. In keeping with DH (1999a) policy regarding qualitative healthcare, services are currently charged, as part of their overall clinical governance role (Secker-Walker and Donaldson 2001), with providing contemporary evidence-based risk assessments that direct care and treatment and reduce risks (Doyle 2000). Any such individual assessment must be facilitated by an awareness of the relevant research knowledge (Grounds 1995). At a basic level, clinicians who identify risks have a responsibility to act so that risks are reduced and effectively managed (Reed 1997). This is what service users want (Manthorpe and Alaszewski 2000; Robert 2006).

However, Higgins *et al.* (2005) found high variability in practice within general adult psychiatry amongst randomly selected trusts across England when reviewing risk assessments in use to manage harm to others. This included both a lack of consensus concerning suitable methods of risk assessment and variance in training availability. Kettles *et al.*'s (2003) review of risk assessment in UK forensic psychiatric units recommended a need for more consistent approaches using both reliable and valid up-to-date tools, on a multidisciplinary basis, which in turn could aid care continuity and individual care pathways. Shortfalls in consistency, reliability and validity in locally designed processes were also emergent findings in MacCall's (2003) forensic risk assessment review of healthcare in Australia and New Zealand, from which he declared a necessity for more robust research to improve efficacy. Similar themes are integral to recent UK national guidelines (DH 2007) for best practice in risk management, which propose that up-to-date evidence bases be embedded in everyday risk management, so that assessment of users' recovery, structured risk assessment, collaborative MDT working and positive risk management become commonplace in mental health services.

Potts (1995) revealed what are perceived as factors found in good risk assessments from a Home Office perspective. These include:

- quality and range of information;
- completeness and objectivity of analysis;
- concrete evidence of progress;
- realistic forward planning.

(See Potts' chapter for a wider expansion of criteria.)

O'Rourke *et al.* (1997) went further with their proposed Risk Assessment Management and Audit System (RAMAS) as a model to help clinicians in their roles in individual care and public safety. RAMAS measures dangerousness, mental instability, self-harm and vulnerability on an MDT basis involving service users. It is aimed at informing risk management strategies and facilitating both structure and support to decision making.

The DH (1995) also articulates that the key principle of risk assessment is to use all available resources of information; otherwise a proper assessment cannot be made. Admittedly, this can be an arduous but nonetheless essential practice, yet as Grounds (1995) claims, thorough risk assessments are resource dependent, particularly taking into account the realities of service pressures. Does this mean that services are likely to be swamped by the ever-competing demands for precious time, which is more noticeable in its absence than its availability amongst MHNs and MDTs? The author suggests that this may be so.

Regardless, in terms of good practice in risk assessment, Holloway (1998) declares a need for balancing the risks and benefits and taking a level of risk that informs patient care decision making, as a product of conservative risk policies can be harmful to patients.

Blumenthal and Lavender (2004, p.118) state:

'Risk assessment does not take place in a vacuum, but is conducted within a socio-political context, which has practical implications both for the outcome of the assessment itself and for the consequences of that assessment in terms of how individuals deemed potentially dangerous are managed.'

It could be argued that the NHS has never been more politically influenced than it is today.

Moore (1996, p.7), in her easy-to-read book *Risk Assessment: A Practitioner's Guide to Predicting Harmful Behaviour*, proposes that a sound risk framework should prompt the following:

- defining the behaviour to be predicted;
- distinguishing between the behaviour's probability and cost;
- having awareness of probable error sources;
- accounting for internal (individual) and external (environmental) issues;
- checking that all required data are collected;
- evaluating when (and if) others need to be involved;
- planning key interventions;
- predicting what is likely to increase/decrease future risks.

From a forensic nursing perspective, Doyle's (2000) seemingly all-encompassing and expansive work (see below for details) on what needs inclusion within that specialty's role can act to inform MHNs of the potential complexities they may face. In addition (p.154), further evidence of potential suitable frameworks is raised. However, many factors alluded to have a capacity to warrant (and quite rightly in many instances) in-depth assessment in their own right. Having cognisance of the past statements about resource dependency and the demands on ever-decreasing available time, MHNs will have to ensure that they retain a sensible balance towards their risk assessment roles, or they may find themselves doing little, if anything, else. In this instance, cognisance is also afforded to the idea that all mental health nursing activities could be construed as risk focused.

Blumenthal and Lavender (2004, p.122), in their work on violence and mental disorder, quote Gunn's (1993) seven-step procedure for risk assessment, which they found useful:

1. Detailed and widely validated personal history.
2. Specific focus on substance misuse and effects.
3. Special attention to sexual interests, attitudes and ideas.
4. Detailed criminal and/or antisocial behaviours.
5. Psychological assessments – intelligence, personality, sexual (if indicated).
6. Mental state assessment over time and events.
7. Descriptors of behaviours, attitudes and responses to treatment.

In addition, Blumenthal and Lavender (2004) recommend adding the following two steps to Gunn's procedure:

- Assessing individuals' social contexts.
- Developing a psychological formulation from the findings above.

Jones and Plowman (2005, p.141) propose that in working towards a gold standard of clinician-based multidisciplinary risk assessment, the minimum on which to base such an assessment should include histories of:

- family background;
- education;
- occupation;
- relationships;
- psychiatric factors;
- substance abuse;
- forensic issues.

A common thread runs through each of these bullet pointed prompts, procedures and proposals, which highlights the need to collect and collate information from as wide a range of sources and agencies as practicably possible. This will obviously be resource dependent, but nevertheless is essential.

Without going into further discussion about definitive frameworks per se, it is important to stress that regardless of what is used, the information needs to be consistently applied by MHNs and, where indicated, by MDTs, so that everyone understands where each other is coming from and what is being aimed at. This should extend to a wide range of agencies, thereby limiting the risk of misinformation and/or vital information going astray (Ireland 2004). This will at least assist in improved communication within and among MDTs and across other professions and agencies (Prins 1999), which has been subject to criticism and projected as warranting further improvement in many of the past Inquiry reports (Holloway 1998; Reith 1998; Robinson *et al.* 2006).

Risk assessment tools

Debate has proliferated and continues around the concepts associated with risk assessment tools. Szmukler (2003) sees the development of tools as a major task, necessitating separate tests within respective populations to enhance precision and accuracy of the tools. Prins (1999) suggests that hindsight would be a good tool when improvements in both risk assessment and management are required. However, he also indicates that there are no statistical or actuarial tools available to deliver certainty in predicting dangerous behaviours in any offenders, though they can distinguish between high-risk and low-risk groups. This may invalidate their use in individual cases. Jones and Plowman (2005, p.135) acknowledge that the availability of actuarial data enriches risk assessment, providing *'an anchor against the force of bias'* where it may exist.

What, if any, actuarial tools should be used is very much driven by the areas in need of assessment. For example, assessment of violence risk might include use of the *HCR-20 Assessing Risk for Violence (Version 2)* (Webster *et al.* 1997) or the Violence Risk Appraisal Guide (VRAG) (Quinsey *et al.* 1998), whilst individuals thought to have psychopathic tendencies may benefit from assessment using the Psychopathy Checklist-Revised (PCL-R) (Hare 1991). Service users with sex offending histories may warrant use of a Sex Offender Risk Appraisal Guide (SORAG) (Quinsey *et al.* 1998) or the Rapid Risk Assessment for Sexual Offence Recidivism (RRASOR) (Hanson 1997) (and cited by Hanson 2004). Similarly, individuals for whom anger is a problem may be the subject of assessment using Spielberger's (1999) *State-Trait Anger Expression Inventory – 2 (STAXI-2)*.

Not wishing to have an extended debate about the validity of these tools, it seems prudent to point out Moore's (1996) claim of it being professionally negligent to use unproven and/or outdated methods when more valid, reliable or ethically better alternatives are available. Similarly, recent work by Hart *et al.* (2007) has commenced debate about the precision of actuarial tools, in this instance two violence actuarial risk assessment instruments, by suggesting that their margins of error for risk estimates were substantial, at both group and individual levels, claiming that from the latter's perspective, their research findings were suggestive that the test results were virtually meaningless. This will no doubt proliferate further discussion and debate about the efficacy of actuarial tools, but they are likely to be in continual use until valid, reliable and substantive consistent evidence emerges concerning their effectiveness.

Much of the expanding work on risk assessment has its background in violence and subsequent links to mental disorder. It is hard to have a definitive view on whether this is connected to the public's exaggerated perceptions of links between the two (Munro and Rumgay 2000), or whether it is because now psychiatry is closer to the general public given United Kingdom (UK) community care policies (Snowden 1997). However, if taking a snapshot from the United States (US), Monahan's (2001) introduction in another influential work entitled *Rethinking Risk Assessment* (Monahan *et al.* 2001) provides food for thought. He claims that despite major developments in diagnosing and treating mental disorders, great social stigma exists for those experiencing such disorders. He cites the US Surgeon General's (1999) first report on mental health, which suggests that fear of violence, particularly associated with those having mental illness, and more significantly psychosis, is a driving force behind and subsequently influences mental health law and policy within the US and worldwide.

Contrastingly, Busfield (2002) proclaims that many UK advocates have argued that those with psychiatric needs are no more likely than those without to engage in violence, and public stereotypes are false. Regardless, Taylor (2001, p.8) indicates, *'There is no longer any doubt that there is an association between some mental disorders and violence, but only a modest one'*, with some degree of collective confirmation across varying studies, with different variables eliciting findings across several disorders.

Hodgins' (2004) description of working with offenders with major mental disorders also implies that there are links between disorder and criminality, including violence, though this may have been impacted upon by policy changes, including more community-based care. She goes on to claim that improvements in prevention could emerge if funding and policy decisions were based on empirical evidence and if treatment programme effectiveness was informed by programme evaluation, thereby improving treatment efficacy.

Although the author acknowledges that a range of evidence will both support and offer counter-arguments and contention to this often emotive yet important issue (Busfield 2002), and that many uncertainties exist, further debate about any suggestive links between the two are beyond the scope of this chapter. Maybe Snowden (1997, p.32) takes a realistic position by stating, *'Risk should not be narrowly equated with violence to others'*.

However, given Prins' (2005b) statement of the government's position over the past decade on public protection, should it not be expected that a focus on violence risk is logical? This may be expected by some, given the current NHS mental health services' and political agendas (Mason 1998; Doyle and Dolan 2002). Similarly, the major NHS thrust towards assessing and managing violence more effectively (National Institute for Mental Health in England 2004a) and a push towards zero tolerance serve to reinforce its importance.

Early work in violence risk assessment used unstructured clinical or professional opinions/judgement factors to inform views on risk (Doyle and Dolan 2002). Within this, Hart (2001) implies that the assessor/evaluator had some discretion in how and what information was collected and decisions made therein. Similarly, he suggested that the process could be characterised as intuitive or experiential, though lacking in empirical basis. Not surprisingly, Monahan's (1981) review on the accuracy of predicting violence using clinical judgement concluded that no more than one in three predictions of violent behaviour made by psychiatrists and psychologists were accurate (cited in Monahan and Steadman 1994).

The subsequent development of actuarial violence risk assessments, despite the time-consuming and effort-driven factors associated with their construction and validation (Hart 2001), still informs current discussions. Although perceived as seemingly superior/better than the unstructured clinical judgement processes discussed above, they still have their drawbacks, in particular their inability to offer wide generalisations of their validity to populations other than those that the said tools have been developed with (Monahan *et al.* 2001).

Munro and Rumgay (2000) comment on the low accuracy of risk assessments, with more empirical research similar to the MacArthur Risk Assessment Study (Steadman *et al.* 1994; and subsequently Monahan *et al.* 2001) necessary. Quinsey *et al.* (1998, p.171) (who developed the VRAG) claimed:

'. . . we are calling on clinicians to do risk appraisal in a new way – a different way in which most of us were trained. What we are advising is not the addition of actuarial methods to existing practice, but rather the complete replacement of existing practice with actuarial methods. . . . Actuarial methods are too good and clinical judgment too poor to risk contaminating the former with the latter.'

No doubt in response to their forceful opinions, they acknowledged their understanding and the appropriateness of both the resistance and scepticism they encountered, validating their views on a need for change. Doyle and Dolan (2002) offer further evidence of the limitations associated with using actuarial methods alone, whilst Monahan *et al.* (2001) suggest that actuarial methods should assist clinical practice, with Douglas and Belfrage (2001) reporting that the HCR-20 (Webster *et al.* 1997) should complement clinical practice, not supplant it.

The notion of combining the two previously mentioned risk assessment processes into 'structured clinical/professional judgement' now seems indicated (Maden 2003). Blumenthal and Lavender (2004, p.79) appear to validate the idea by suggesting:

'The dichotomising of actuarial and clinical approaches to risk assessment, in which clinical approach has been equated with subjective judgement, has been unhelpful. A thorough assessment of each actuarial risk factor requires expert clinical judgement. Insights gained using clinical impressions provide important information which is useful in planning the management of risk.'

Hart (2001) also implies support for this principle, highlighting the HCR-20 (Version 2) (Webster *et al.* 1997) as an example. Contained within are attempts to define considered risks; define what information should be gathered and how; and identify the comprehensive core risk factors, drawn from the evidence base and proposed as enhancing consistency, usefulness and the transparency of decision-making. Kennedy (2001) reports that clinical judgements and prediction are contextual and subject to review based on information drawn from patients' and clinicians' experiences, and, as such, are not made in a statistically pure vacuum.

A need for risk training

Whilst examining lessons learnt from then recent inquiries, Reed (1997) articulated that many failures needed and would benefit from multiprofessional and multiagency training. Similarly, Moss and Paice (2001) advocate risk management training for healthcare professionals on a multiprofessional basis, so that errors created via professional gaps, despite professionals working together, can be minimised. The notion of training gains additional support from Higgins *et al.*'s (2005) findings that within their general adult psychiatry sample, around half the psychiatry units provided training in risk assessment, although many consultants did not attend. Whether this validates Moss and Paice's (2001) views of medical education being isolated, tribal and hierarchical is questionable.

By contrast, Petch (2001) states that no amount of risk assessment and management training, whether high quality or not, will make an impact if mental health services are not well resourced. If resources emerge, he claims that risk improvements will follow.

The *National Confidential Inquiry* (DH 1999b) also recommended the need for staff training in relation to those who had contact with patients at risk of suicide. Components of that training are articulated as risk recognition, assessment and management initiatives focused on both suicide and violence. Training was perceived as being required at no longer than 3-yearly intervals.

A similar proposal was recommended in the *National Suicide Prevention Strategy for England* (DH 2002b). The focused strategy detailed within the *Dual Diagnosis Good Practice Guide* (DH 2002a) highlights the need for interagency training, within which risk assessment and management are integral components. Key principles are also addressed towards linking risk assessment and management to mental health, alcohol and drug factors. Moreover, differences in risk and protective factors in the mental health of women and men need recognition as a training development necessity within the implementation guide *Mainstreaming Gender and Women's Mental Health* (DH 2003).

Additionally, given that service users are seen as *'experts by experience'* (National Institute for Mental Health in England 2004a, p.11), national strategies are increasingly reinforcing that service users and their carers/ families become involved in training on a more regular basis. Risk is no exception.

The Standing Nursing and Midwifery Advisory Committee (SNMAC) (1999) highlighted that, as part of the safe and supportive observation of patients at risk, the assessment of risk should form an integral part of the training packages linked to this initiative. Managing risk best practice guidelines (DH 2007) also validates the need for relevant multidisciplinary training updated at not less than 3-yearly intervals.

In terms of HCR-20 use, the designers (Webster *et al.* 1997) recommend that those undertaking assessments have expertise in conducting individual assessments, as in order to administer and interpret findings, considerable professional skill and judgement is required. Recent specifically focused HCR-20 training undertaken by the author and a cohort of nearly 40 MDT colleagues from a UK medium-secure unit has been seen as the very first step in enabling the service to utilise risk assessment as its preferred risk template. An outcome has included the drafting of an intended operational plan to roll out the assessment's use by:

- proposing a timetable for the introduction of the HCR-20 assessment for new admissions;
- planning a graded expansion of assessments for current service users, in keeping with their CPA process;
- ensuring that all risk assessments are undertaken by at least two different MDT members;
- enabling regular updates to the minimum standard of at least every 6 months (in keeping with CPAs);
- options for other updates based on need or risk changes;
- planned discussion around expanding training opportunities for more MDT members;
- piloting HCR-20 usage across each of the six MDT teams to analyse effectiveness and enable consistency.

A nearly universally reported outcome from the informative and much-valued training is that those charged with completing risk assessments are very much novices and require guidance and support to both complete and interpret emerging risk data. This will obviously take resources and effort, as experience cannot be gained by anything other than practice and time, but it is a move in the right direction. The teams are under no illusions about this, and see the foreseeable journey as a significant learning curve. Admittedly, one-off training will not be the 'be all and end all' of this process, but it fits nicely with Snowden's (1997) view that there needs to be an amalgam of taught sessions and 'apprenticeship' to enhance the 'risk approach' in clinical practice. A similar standpoint is proposed by Ogloff (2001).

From the perspective of MHNs, given their explicit role in patient risk assessment as detailed in *The Chief Nursing Officer's Review of Mental Health Nursing* (DH 2006), such forms of training are fundamental, given the likelihood that few MHNs will have undergone dedicated training that equips them well enough to engage fully in the risk process generally.

Moore (1996) highlights her development and facilitation of specific risk assessment training programmes, for both mental health and criminal justice workers, from which she has gained improved personal insights from course participants. This seems to suggest that many individuals in practice areas where risk assessment and management have a role to play have the capacity to contribute to expanding everyday working practices and understanding of the breadth and width that risk as a concept demands, without necessarily undertaking formal research to do so. The importance of experiential learning and any on-the-job training initiatives should not be underestimated in this process.

Dedicated training in the use of specific actuarial tools is also essential (Maden 2005), but would necessitate a multidisciplinary attendance so that the uniqueness attributable to each professional group's judgements can be transferred into the greater whole, once risk assessment starts on this basis. This can aid the diversity that will thus emerge from risk assessment, as well as increase objective scrutiny (Jones and Plowman 2005).

MHNs' risk assessment and management roles

Prins (2005b) suggests that there is no doubt that many professionals' risk assessment and management work is high quality, though he also acknowledges past shortfalls. MHNs are an integral part of this professional group and therefore deserve credit. For those shortfalls, MHNs collectively have to work harder. Moreover, as part of the multidisciplinary team functioning that is essential for risk assessment and management (Jones and Plowman 2005), MHNs must ensure that they act in the best interests of service users, use their knowledge, skills and competence, but also realise that they remain accountable for their practices (UKCC 1998).

Frontline MHNs may be far better placed to carry out risk assessments than other multiprofessional colleagues, so long as they are given guidance, and as key professionals they could have access to many of the facts to assess risk (Moore 1996). However, this does not replace but adds to multidisciplinary risk assessment and management.

It is also acknowledged that MHNs are likely to have both diverse and, depending on where they are employed, different operational methods for similar functioning. This is to be expected, given likely service users' needs within different environments such as the community, assertive outreach teams, general adult psychiatry, old-age psychiatry, child and young person mental health services, learning disability nursing, private sector care, Her Majesty's Prisons, and low, medium and high secure facilities, where forensic mental health nurses will be evident. However, given the findings from *The Chief Nursing Officer's Review* (DH 2006), commonalties should exist in each of these and other varied nursing roles.

Doyle (2000) offers an informative perspective on a staged way forward enabling MHNs to facilitate their roles in relation to risk. Although contained within a book for forensic mental health nurses, it is recommended that MHNs may benefit from accessing the book and using it as an aide-memoire for future reference. He makes a useful link between his proposed risk management cycle and the CPA process. The risk management cycle (p.143) includes:

- identification;
- risk assessment;
- risk rating;
- implementation of risk management measures;
- monitoring risk management measures;
- risk assessment review.

As can be alluded to from the above, the involvement of MHNs in risk processes is likely to be cyclic, in the sense that each of the components has an interdependency on the other for risk management processes to be complete and more importantly to meet service users' needs. There is a likelihood of service users identifying new risk factors as improved understanding of them occurs within teams (Hollin 1997). This needs feeding back into the risk cycle.

The author proposes that Doyle's cycle:

- is not only useful but also transferable to most, if not all, MHN environments;
- has the capacity to inform and fit in with those risk practices MHNs are working with; and if not
- at the very least offers a sound framework on which to base nursing practice.

However, cognisance is also given to the previously noted issues concerning resource dependency and service pressures (Grounds 1995).

Recognition is also given to another forensic nursing article (Bowring-Lossock 2006), which offers a thoughtful review of the current status of the role of forensic nursing. Its suggestion that, in order to meet complex and multifaceted service user needs, role development is essential achieves much affinity with that of MHNs. Simplistically, this should be expected, given that many, though not exclusively all, to whom the article applies will be MHNs, although some are likely to have undertaken specialised forensic post-basic education. This could be at a high academic level. MHNs may also have some of the competence, knowledge, skills and personal qualities detailed within the article, and without seeing a resume here are advised to evaluate it of their own volition.

Similarly, a number of associated worthwhile forensic nursing books (including Chaloner and Coffey 2000; Mercer *et al.* 2000; Robinson and Kettles 2000; Dale *et al.* 2001) are worth reviewing.

The conclusions to be drawn from this sojourn into forensic nursing are that:

- there are many overlaps between the two nursing roles;
- knowledge and skills developed over time are transferable;
- MHNs without forensic experience may see efficacy in accessing the aforementioned books as part of their continued personal development;
- risk assessment and management is not solely limited to forensic services.

In relation to the latter, it has been suggested that general psychiatrists manage the largest group of mentally disordered offenders, particularly those who may be about to offend (Holloway 1997).

MHNs who actively pursue service user engagement and managing risks together, as opposed to it being a one-sided activity, improve partnership working and will ultimately improve benefits to users, professionals and the public (Manthorpe and Alaszewski 2000; Robert 2006). However, the author acknowledges that there may be occasions when this is not possible one hundred percent of the time, particularly if crises occur and service users' decision making fails or becomes flawed, which results in needs having to be managed instantly. This can include cases of heightened deliberate self-harm or suicidal or violent behaviours. However, it is proposed that having a milieu in all professional relationships that is non-judgmental, supportive, promotes empowerment, engagement and involvement, and is accepting of criticism, where necessary, may act as a medium through which service users want to have ownership of and responsibility for their actions. The principles and fundamentals of this being subscribed to by all nursing and ultimately MDT members should not require reinforcement here. This may ultimately lead to proactive risk processes.

From an inpatient perspective, one medium that can assist risk assessment and management is that of 'therapeutic security'. Evolving at Rampton Hospital (one of England's high-security hospitals), it is proposed as:

'The management of risk to provide a safe working and living environment where the primary objective of rehabilitation can be achieved. In addition to physical and procedural measures, such security depends on all staff developing constructive relationships with their colleagues and patients, a commitment to therapeutic activity and the provision of safeguards based on the level of risk presented by individual patients. Therapeutic security is a dynamic rather than a static process. It allows the highest quality multidisciplinary approach to care and treatment of patients whilst protecting society's wider interests' (Elvins 1989).

The importance attributed to therapeutic security is that it enables the relational and interpersonal element of service user–MDT interactions to act as the driver through which risk assessment, taking and management initiatives can be maximised, with the confidence that if required any physical and procedural components are already integrated into working philosophies.

Contrastingly, and almost contradictorily, it is also accepted that within psychiatric inpatient aggression, associated diverse clinical, situational and psychological variables that impact on these scenarios, together with certain situational, clinical and demographic characteristics are likely to be present (Daffern and Howells 2002). These have the capacity to impact on specific aggressive episodes. Admittedly, they may not have relevance for every service user individually; but they could have some commonalities both for individuals and within groups, be situation- or person-specific, or show no connectivity whatsoever to different events. Regardless, their presence could no doubt be generalised to the community and other environments. MHNs have to be conscious of and ready to deal with these issues as they emerge, with the minimum amount of detrimental effect to the service user and others.

Given the frontline nature of MHNs' roles, their responsibilities will include working with service users to build up a clinical risk picture that serves to inform future risk management and taking. This is particularly important in areas where harm to others and/or service users themselves could be outcomes. Such activity and experiences serve to add to the role diversity of MHNs, at the same time forming an integral yet key part of their contributions to the risk cycle, supplementing their involvement in improving service user outcomes and recovery (National Institute for Mental Health in England 2004b); but this may also make excessive demands on their time. Part of their overall role functioning therefore includes managing time effectively.

Furthermore, an essential component of the risk assessment and management role of MHNs is their knowledge, skills and expertise in communication. Collins (2000) proclaims that forming a nurse–patient relationship, and the associated skills to achieve this, is a core psychiatric nursing skill. This must take into account both verbal and non-verbal skills, reinforced by heightened knowledge of the effects of communication, particularly its focus and potential outcomes. Admittedly, this has an impact in all that MHNs do, but its necessity, essentiality and effectiveness cannot be understated when its focus is risk-based. The importance of MHNs communicating honestly and with clarity, together with being receptive and empathic listeners (Clarke 2006), cannot be overemphasised.

Cordall (1999) reported that the following clinical skills are also essential:

- taking time to gain trust;
- acting as an enabler;
- being reliable and consistent;
- listening to and hearing what is said;
- maintaining boundaries;
- achieving disclosure.

Each must be MHN characteristics. To validate their importance, it is proposed that many MHNs will have little difficulty in reflecting on where others, or indeed themselves, have either made mistakes, said the wrong thing at the wrong time, thereby exacerbating risk behaviours, or not said the right thing at the right time to limit or manage events, likely being linked to service users harming others or themselves. This should not be perceived as criticism of the profession, but should be accepted from the perspective that everyone makes mistakes. Many learn from them, after self-reflection and/or guidance from others. It is near impossible to predict most things correctly, but consequences have the potential to be severe. Past inquiries abound (see discussion above; e.g. Reith 1998) where communication shortfalls have lead to tragedy. It would be welcoming to suggest that these issues become less problematic the more educated and experienced professionals become, but this may not necessarily be the case (see Robinson *et al.* 2006 for further validation).

More specifically, in terms of communicating risk assessment results (although focused towards HCR-20 assessments, but having just as much validity for any communication) Webster *et al.* (1997) highlight the need for such reports to be written so that misinterpretation by readers (in this instance courts, review boards, parole boards, etc.) is minimised. This is just as vital when formulating written communication for distribution both within and outwith teams and to other agencies. Inaccuracies here may create significant problems for service users further on in their contact with respective services. Communicating risk reports effectively is also perceived by Ireland (2004) as being vitally important, particularly for its actual and potential implications on service users, victims and the professionals involved. A responsibility therefore rests with individuals in the first instance, and MDTs secondly, to ensure that risks are communicated effectively and as widely as required.

Communication by MHNs cannot take place without intrapersonal factors impacting on experiences. For instance, Cordall (1999) reported that MHNs' self-awareness of particularly their attitudes, beliefs and feelings, and having an 'us and them' mentality, had an impact on how angry women mentally disordered offenders were managed. It is proposed that similar criteria can impinge on MHNs' risk activity also. Therefore, MHNs need to have both self-confidence and openness to acknowledge the existence of potentially counter-therapeutic self-perceptions (Schultz and Videbeck 2005) in relation to risk, more specifically any service user risk factor, so that they can be minimised, and any biased impact that might be detrimental to their role can be eliminated. Service users will benefit from MHNs positioning themselves accordingly (Robert 2006).

At a similar level, MHNs' commitment to and engagement in recognition skills and observational behaviours also complement their risk roles (Standing Nursing and Midwifery Advisory Committee 1999; National Institute for Mental Health in England 2004a). Such actions may be of greater importance when MHNs are seeing service users for short periods of time, with long periods between appointments such as outpatient clinics or in users' homes. Having recognition and observational skills and the clinical acumen associated with them may make a significant difference in preventing or managing a potential risk effectively, as opposed to leaving service users in crisis, at risk, with heightened vulnerability or one simple step away from major adversity. Not to undervalue the simplicity, yet essentiality, of observation and recognition skills in the risk process is a key message (SNMAC 1999). This may meet mental health services' dual commitment to public protection and service user welfare (Munro and Rumgay 2000). However, this is not to state the seemingly obvious, but rather to propose that this recognition remains a central tenet of MHN risk activity. Whether or not influenced by policies and/or procedures, or forming part of defined clinical pathways or guidelines (Foy *et al.* 2001), recognition and observational skills remain essential components within the complexities of the Clinical Negligence Scheme for Trusts (Walshe 2001).

Ultimately, the reason MHNs engage in observation is to enhance service user outcomes, but also to improve accuracy should incidents occur that necessitate reports (Secker-Walker and Taylor-Adams 2001). Admittedly, observation can be exceedingly resource draining on already-highlighted service pressures, often to the detriment of other MHN activities.

Occasionally they can be monotonous or demotivating for individuals, but unfortunately, until something, if anything, evolves or research suggests that observation makes no difference in managing risk, the nursing profession will continue to fulfil this role most of the time.

One salient point to make, however, is that it should not be common practice for service users to be placed on increased levels of observation as a matter of course whilst within inpatient care, simply to manage risks (National Institute for Mental Health in England 2004a). This needs to be based on need and/or drawn from known past risks when in previous similar positions. A question to reflect on in this context is: 'How are community-based or outpatient service users' risks managed?' They are unlikely to be provided with enhanced or special observations, despite being exposed to potentially more risks. From an opposite perspective, it also seems vital to reveal that, in some instances, heightened levels of observation, close monitoring and surveillance are required that goes beyond that which is the norm (Prins 2005a). In what circumstances this takes place is likely to be determined by those MHNs (without other MDT colleagues during initial decision making in many instances) who have developed risk expertise and experiences on which to draw from. This can be informed by accurate past records of previous behaviours.

Additionally, teamwork within MDTs is vital. Traditionally, nurses have played a subservient and/or limited role therein when compared to other colleagues (Prins 1999), but now, even more to the fore given their roles in risk, they are expected to and have an equal role to undertake in risk assessment, taking and management processes. Their involvement will contribute to the team's decision making and enhance change (Antrobus 1998). Their impact will be influenced by many variables. From the author's perspective, these could include:

- having a valued voice;
- being integrated within the team itself;
- sharing common goals;
- showing commonsense;
- proving that background work has been done and risk awareness is evident.

However, the role of MHNs in contributing to the team's impetus and coherence generally (Byalin 1989; Landrum *et al.* 2000; Chambers *et al.* 2001) remains essential. This must include supporting the development of the team (Alimo-Metcalfe and Alban-Metcalfe 2000).

Teamwork involvement is also influenced by risk assessment activity being multidisciplinary in nature, given the impossibility of one individual accessing and/or retaining requisite risk assessment information (Jones and

Plowman 2005). Importantly, risk processes are not reconciled with those who want to go it alone or be prima donnas (Prins 2005b), as a team's success is bound by each individual contributing to the process having an equal position and status. Past Inquiry reports (e.g. Robinson *et al.* 2006) have highlighted where this has not been the case.

Additionally, given their position, and if only by the amount of time they spend with service users by comparison with other members of the team, particularly in inpatient settings, MHNs are often those who are exposed to the potential problems or risk incidents as they are about to occur and/or as new risk evidence emerges. These can include dealing with immediate face to face issues such as violence, deliberate self-harm, abuse of others, absconding, property damage or exacerbation of mental health problems. Not only do MHNs, when faced with any of these or other risk issues, need an array of crisis management skills to deal with such, but also they require an explicit conscious self-understanding and self-efficacy that they have the MDT's support behind them, for what can often be a split-second decision. Within this short time frame they have to act both intuitively and with forethought to achieve a safe conclusion from what can be very challenging scenarios, with service users' best interests at the forefront of their intentions.

As previously referred to, the majority of those decisions have no adverse long-lasting effects, but MHNs are not infallible, just like their colleagues. When events take place that no one could foresee or when risk assessment and taking initiatives have been worked through to meet the service user's needs in a specific way and then go horribly wrong, as they inevitably can do, some initial comfort and understanding might be taken from MHNs' conscious knowledge that they were acting as part of a wider team, as opposed to alone. This is not to condone inappropriateness, incompetence or acts of stupidity, but rather to give MDTs and ultimately trusts shared responsibility and accountability for risks taken (Secker-Walker and Donaldson 2001).

Having explicit reference within trusts that they operate a just culture, as opposed to one of blame, will go some way to ensuring that MHN and MDT risk taking practices do not become risk averse, which would be contradictory to clinical governance initiatives. Risk assessment and management must be founded on both evidence-based and safe practice. This does not mean that trusts will take the concept of risk lightly and undermine their own clinical risk management schemes, but rather it means that they will send the appropriate messages that support is available for staff who have acted responsibly and defensibly where risks have occurred, but that their prevention cannot be guaranteed (Kemshall 1999). If trusts take a position of this nature, then on a macro level a just culture appears clear. It would be welcomed even further if that was recognised within socio-political environments of central government and by the public itself. However, on a more micro basis, this may simply take the form of:

- having regular MDT meetings to assess and evaluate current risk activity;
- sharing presenting problems within and amongst MDTs preferably or within unidisciplinary events;
- engaging in risk planning initiatives;
- simple problem-solving.

Integral to MHNs' risk activities is the need for clinical supervision and support. Collins (2000) highlights that MHNs have their own set of thoughts, feelings and moral values, but are often seen as 'bullet-proof' individuals, taking anything thrown at them. Though they are not human sponges (far from it), they will require a chance to offload. Clinical supervision facilitates this process (Kohner 1994). Clear distinction needs to be made between clinical supervision and management supervision, although it is acknowledged that confusion does exist between the two (Yegdich 1999). The former is classed as something that MHNs have a degree of electivity about, not whether they engage or not, but in a sense of who their clinical supervisor may be. From personal experience, it also enables a 'safe environment' in which to disclose information. The latter is likely to involve an MHN's immediate line manager, which, although an essential activity, is likely to have different objectives as its focus, being a more mandatory practice, potentially perceived as threatening by the supervisee, and with more negativity and suspicion by comparison therein (Shanley and Stevenson 2006).

Individual supervision is usually integrated into MHNs' everyday practice, both as part of the operational policies of a trust and from its recognition as essential to aiding reflection in order to improve service user recovery (DH 2006). Within these parameters it is vital that MHNs both access and use supervision to evaluate any of their perceived shortfalls, and also plan and explore options that will aid their development and monitor these at regular intervals. Part of this process might include having somebody other than a nurse as a clinical supervisor, which can add another multidisciplinary dimension to the supervisory process. This follows the line that if risk is a multidisciplinary process, then why can't supervision and guidance targeted at such come from a multidisciplinary colleague? To the author's knowledge, there is nothing concrete to say that it cannot.

Part of the wider supervisory process is the use of preceptorship for newly qualified MHNs or MHNs new to the working environment (Nursing and Midwifery Council (NMC) 2003), although it has been reported that preceptorship has been incorporated into clinical supervision (Shanley and Stevenson 2006). The author proposes that for the new MHN, preceptorship will have a similar function to what it fulfils for students – enabling coping with uncertainty and exploring fears of the unknown (Charleston and Happel 2005), as well as generally supporting role development. The NMC also proclaims that it can be invaluable for all new nurses and those having had career gaps, in order to gain support and guidance from a more experienced nurse in the early phases of their career. It strongly advocates that preceptorship should occur over a defined period (about 4 months in the NMC's view), but does not abdicate the preceptee from his or her own responsibilities and subsequent accountability.

MHNs who act as preceptors should display behaviours that are seen as enabling to students, so it follows that MHNs should continue to utilise similar behaviours with new staff. These include showing attitudes, behaviours and support that are welcoming, nurturing and inclusive so that new staff can relax and learn more; thus helping the application of knowledge and skills and acting as a resource for professional development (Nursing and Midwifery Council 2003; Charleston and Happel 2005). Making these commodities available and having them in the skills repertoire of MHNs is a major addition to risk processes generally.

The contributions of MHNs when engaged in therapeutic activity with service users – whether it be something as simple as one-to-one communication, playing a game, involvement in leisure pursuits, or the more dynamic, though not necessarily more important, work of counselling or treating problems and needs through specific individual or group treatments (Hollin 2004) – are invaluable. It is not uncommon for new risk evidence to be found in these circumstances (as previously mentioned), and the notion of engagement does much to retain up-to-date and contemporary inside views of service users' thoughts, feelings and behaviours. This must not be perceived as something underhand or sneaky, but, based on the previous discussed positioning of empowering service users to have greater responsibility for their risks, contributes to enabling service users to take that responsibility and learn lessons from issues that emerge accordingly. Anecdotally, health-care support workers, given their closeness to everyday service user activity, are often a vital source of risk information; and with nurturing and on-the-job training from MHNs to improve their knowledge and skills bases, they can add much to treatment continuums and ultimately risk assessment and management. They must not be undervalued in any way.

A key to meeting risk needs, as part of this process, revolves around MHNs' involvement with and use of dedicated care plans. These may include:

- evidence-based individual nursing plans (Neilson *et al.* 1996) focusing on specific nurse-led initiatives;
- plans that have been designed in collaboration with MDTs as part of the risk continuum (Schultz and Videbeck 2005);

- wider-based treatment plans, usually MDT focused but not necessarily drawn up by MHNs.

The latter includes substantial treatment programmes that meet definitive service user needs, for example anger (Novaco 1975), problem solving skills (McGuire 2001) and sex offenders (Marshall 2004).

The influence that nursing care plans bring to clinical practice cannot be stressed highly enough. This is because they (as informed by Schultz and Videbeck 2005, p.4):

- provide a focus for deliberate nursing process use with service users;
- provide the basis to evaluate nursing intervention effectiveness and enable care plan revision, as opposed to unspecific or haphazard intervention;
- are the only feasible means of effective and increased communication about service user care among varying nursing staff;
- provide centrality for care coordination information, objectives of care, any limits used, interventions and evaluations;
- maintain consistency and continuity in each care environment;
- are required to meet nursing care standards and accreditation standards;
- facilitate efficient care that saves time and avoids staff burnout;
- avoid repetition, particularly when practice needs changing (what has gone on previously will be evident).

Additionally, care plans assist MHNs and student nurses to learn, and whilst providing a defensible document on which to base nursing practice, they articulate appropriate evidence base use by MHNs. Additionally, they act as media through which resources for nursing activity can be argued, and offer definitive reasons why qualified nurses are essential for service users to achieve the optimum level of contemporary care they duly deserve and are expecting in today's NHS.

The input of MHNs in each of these initiatives will facilitate expanding their knowledge and skills bases, particularly when contributing to improving what they know about what works and with whom. Whether or not this evolves to MHNs contributing to the multidisciplinary research process at the same time (Thompson 2000) remains to be seen. Admittedly, MHNs engaging in research and audit have received little cognisance within the scope of this chapter, but nonetheless the importance of research and audit must not be forgotten or undervalued.

Robinson and Collins (1999) reported care planning (and therefore care plans) as a powerful model to document, provide and evaluate service user care in a systematic way, which ultimately can contribute to expanding the evidence base, but they were also critical of it, particularly concerning factors linked to ill-equipped assessment models and the variability with which individuals had taken account of it as a concept. However, the author takes something of a different perspective in as much that although care plans will only be as good as those MHNs writing them, it is the ownership of them by service users and MHNs alike that will give them the credence they deserve.

It is up to the leaders of MHNs to ensure that care plans are used to inform what they should do, that they are guided by validated evidence bases, and that clinical practice is founded on them, not continued simply through tradition and myth. The care plan is something that can validate the role of MHNs in these times of financial prudence, but only if they grasp the concepts of evidence-based practice and show that they can use it. When MDTs use contemporary evidence, service users should get the best possible care, but the uniqueness of each professional's role and skills will complement a range of issues that service users can draw upon (Forchuk 2001). However, it is also acknowledged that there remains no magic wand to make healthcare evidence based (Tomlin *et al.* 2002).

For MHNs to develop their risk processes they need to be leaders and require leadership. Individually and within their groups the author thinks that they need to show a mix of leadership values, skills and behaviours. However, they may also be faced with the dilemma of having the burden and privilege to challenge boundaries that others never think to question (Berwick 1998). From a risk perspective this could be good and contribute to its management, though Berwick also places a rider to challenges in indicating that only a fool tries to achieve the impossible.

Leadership attitudes that MHNs need include issues such as having self-awareness, which has significance with regard to their capacity to become effective leaders (Gunden and Crissman 1992; Alimo-Metcalfe 1998), though this must be linked to others' views of themselves also. Key components include:

- MHNs being service user driven (Perkins 1996);
- enabling users to have choice through informed consent (Pilgrim 1997);
- improving users' health outcomes and recovery (Turner-Crowson and Wallcraft 2002).

For leadership skills to be successful they need to be empowering (Rae 2000), increase autonomy (Gunden and Crissman 1992) and enable everyone to help improve (Berwick 1998). Displaying exceptional communication skills and vision (Easton 2002), promoting direction finding and decision making (Collier and Esteban 2000), and having and using political astuteness (Malby 1998; Alimo-Metcalfe 1999) remain vital. The ability to display and use teaching, coaching and role modelling skills (Brown 2002) cannot be understated. It is essential in providing dedicated on-the-job risk training, and also acts as a framework for training the experienced MHNs of the future. Perhaps some of the key cornerstones in respect of leadership skills include thinking creatively and analytically (Alimo-Metcalfe and Alban-Metcalfe 2000), having self-belief (Howell and Avolio 1993) and celebrating the success of others (Clegg 2000). The author thinks that the latter is not done frequently enough.

Contrastingly, leadership behaviours used are likely to:

- be those MHNs are comfortable with (Landrum *et al.* 2000);
- involve developing their own style, drawn from both transformational and transactional models (Alimo-Metcalfe 1999);
- inspire shared visions;
- challenge thinking;
- encourage flexibility and innovation (Easton 2002);
- remain transparent throughout (Hackett *et al.* 1999).

Change must not be shied away from.

More significantly, leadership behaviours that shape the future of mental health nursing (Benner 2000) but also health policy and practice (Antrobus and Kitson 1999) are viewed by the author as a fundamental component for all MHNs to subscribe to, regardless of experience and seniority, as it is MHNs who hold the future of mental health nursing in their hands, and ultimately the future of service users, carers and families.

The emphasis that has been given to MHNs' leadership as opposed to management is based on the notion that how nurses apply their leadership repertoire has the capacity to greatly inform risk assessment and management from a nursing perspective. This is not undermining or devaluing management. However, in today's NHS culture of engagement, facilitation, partnerships, service user choice and the changes that these have brought about, transformational leadership has been viewed as more in tune with its contemporary needs (Ewens 2002). It seems more related to risk's fluidity. However it is vital that management is not forgotten in the risk process, as it can have just as influential a role, if managers move from the traditions of bureaucratic and hierarchical influences (Dale *et al.* 2002) to having a blend of functional management and leadership behaviours. Admittedly, transactional behaviours are still required, but not at the expense of transformational leadership roles (Alimo-Metcalfe 1999). This may not be possible without some shift in managers' functioning, yet whether this can be done easily or remains an unlikely possibility in today's management era of targets and monitoring begs another debate.

Conclusion

The notion that the risk assessment, taking and management agendas continue to place demands on MHNs and mental health services is unquestionable and, as such, they will continue to do so for the foreseeable future, particularly in the current socio-political climate of high priority for public protection. Admittedly, from service users' perspectives this has to be balanced with both meeting their needs and aiding their recovery. This creates a dilemma and whether the two are currently balanced is worthy of further debate and the discussion will no doubt continue.

The need for MHNs, MDTs and trusts alike to ensure that their everyday practice in service user care and treatment and clinical risk management play a significant part in contributing to the risk agenda remains paramount. It is proposed that taking gambles with risk in any part is tantamount to precipitating and increasing the likelihood of subsequent inquiry. This is not what services and their users, carers and families want, but sometimes it is inevitable, as past inquiries have seen.

If MHNs, their MDT colleagues and service users collaborate on the basis that each has to understand the other in terms of risk concepts, possibly through sharing a common language, then opportunity for service users to take greater responsibility for their risks may precipitate some risk reduction. However, this may not be a wholesale shift and, as has been stated above, cannot be guaranteed. The premise of 'tolerability' as opposed to 'acceptability' in the sense of risks, particularly if and when something goes wrong, must be at the centre of all decision making. This should inform a just culture as opposed to one of blame where risk assessment and management might become risk averse. Service users do not want the latter. Messages must also be forthcoming that professionals cannot be expected to get it right every time, just as society itself does not. This is not suggesting they abdicate their risk responsibilities, far from it, but there is a sharp contrast between undertaking their professional obligations in a defensible manner, informed by appropriate evidence, and guaranteeing their success one hundred percent.

There are risk assessment tools that teams may use to complement their clinical practice, not supplant it. If they are shown to contribute to more structured clinical judgement, services will benefit. Admittedly, there are concerns about their efficacy, but until healthcare services have used them, how will they know? It remains unlikely that there will ever be a utopian risk assessment and management tool that suits all. Something is better than nothing and will be expected if things go wrong. Part of MHNs' activity could include validating the tools' effectiveness within their MDT, thereby shaping clinical judgement.

National strategy documents and guidelines abound with risk-related issues, along with proposals to train staff to meet them. This may not always be that easy to achieve, given what seem ever-increasing demands on MHNs and healthcare services. It is perceived that multidisciplinary and multi-agency training are the best exemplars in terms of the development of MDTs, which promulgates a notion of shared responsibility for risk. This needs maximising and must not be left to one or two disciplines.

From an MHN's perspective, a number of key, though not exhaustive, attitudes, knowledge and skills are proposed, though these are just a small part of what should complement wider everyday mental health nursing risk practices. MHNs' clinical acumen to use such skills in times of crises is not undervalued by MDTs, and as such their capacity to contribute to risk debates is already cemented in their practice. Resting on laurels is not an option, as continuous service improvements focusing on service user risks remain. Options that may help professional development are also recommended.

It is perhaps apt that the final word is left to the wisdom of Prins (2002) – *'risk is a risky business'*.

References

Alaszewski, A. (1998) Risk in modern society. In: *Risk, Health and Welfare* (eds A. Alaszewski, L. Harrison & J. Manthorpe), pp 3–23. Open University Press, Buckingham.

Alimo-Metcalfe, B. (1998) 360 Degree feedback and leadership development. *International Journal of Selection and Assessment*, **6**(1), 35–44.

Alimo-Metcalfe, B. (1999) Leadership in the NHS: what are the competencies and qualities needed and how can they be developed? In: *Organisational Behaviour in Health Care* (eds L.M. Annabelle & S. Dopson), pp 135–151. Macmillan Business, Basingstoke.

Alimo-Metcalfe, B. & Alban-Metcalfe, R. (2000) Heaven can wait. *Health Service Journal*, **12**, 26–29.

Antrobus, S. (1998) Thoroughly modern leaders. *Nursing Times*, **94**(18), 66–67.

Antrobus, S. & Kitson, A. (1999) Nursing leadership: influencing and shaping health policy and nursing practice. *Journal of Advanced Nursing*, **29**(3), 746–753.

Benner, P. (2000) Shaping the future of nursing. *Nursing Management*, **7**(1), 31–35.

Berwick, D.M. (1998) Crossing the boundary: changing mental models in the service of improvement. *International Journal for Quality in Health Care*, **10**(5), 435–441.

Bingley, W. (1997) Assessing dangerousness: protecting the interests of patients. *British Journal of Psychiatry*, **170**(32), 28–29.

Blumenthal, S. & Lavender, T. (2004) *Violence and Mental Disorder: A Critical Aid to the Assessment and Management of Risk*. Jessica Kingsley, London.

Bowring-Lossock, E. (2006) The forensic mental health nurse – a literature review. *Journal of Psychiatric and Mental Health Nursing*, **13**(6), 780–785.

Brown, M. (2002) *Developing Coaching Skills and Asking Powerful Questions*. Paper presented to National Mental Health Nursing Leadership Programme, York, January. Personal Lecture Notes.

Busfield, J. (2002) Psychiatric disorder and individual violence: imagined death, risk and mental health policy. In: *Care of the Mentally Disordered Offender in the Community* (ed. A. Buchanan), pp 65–88. Oxford University Press, Oxford.

Byalin, K. (1989) Managing to win: front-line leadership in public mental health settings. *Administration and Policy in Mental Health*, **16**(4), 191–198.

Chaloner, C. & Coffey, M. (eds) (2000) *Forensic Mental Health Nursing: Current Approaches*. Blackwell Science, Oxford.

Chambers, R., Boath, E. & Wakely, G. (2001) Clinical governance and mental healthcare. In: *Mental Healthcare Matters in Primary Care* (eds R. Chambers, E. Boath & G. Wakely), pp 1–25. Radcliffe Medical Press, Oxon.

Charleston, R. & Happel, B. (2005) Coping with uncertainty within the preceptorship of students: the perceptions of nursing students. *Journal of Psychiatric and Mental Health Nursing*, **12**(3), 303–309.

Clarke, C. (2006) Relating with professionals. *Journal of Psychiatric and Mental Health Nursing*, **13**, 522–526.

Clegg, A. (2000) Leadership: improving the quality of patient care. *Nursing Standard*, **14**(30), 43–45.

Collier, J. & Esteban, R. (2000) Systemic leadership: ethical and effective. *The Leadership and Organisational Development Journal*, **21**(4), 207–215.

Collins, M. (2000) The practitioner new to the role of forensic psychiatric nurse in the UK. In: *Forensic Nursing and Multidisciplinary Care of the Mentally Disordered Offender* (eds D. Robinson & A. Kettles), pp 39–50. Jessica Kingsley, London.

Cooke, D. (2007) *Violence Risk Assessment: Structured Clinical Judgement Approaches*. Training presented to the Yorkshire Centre for Forensic Psychiatry, Wakefield, May. Lecture and Personal Notes.

Cordall, J. (1999) Angry women mentally disordered offenders: a need to do more? *British Journal of Nursing*, **8**(10), 658–663.

Crowe, M. (2003) Deconstructing risk assessment and management in mental health nursing (issues and innovations in nursing practice). *Journal of Advanced Nursing*, **43**(1), 19–27.

Daffern, M. & Howells, K. (2002) Psychiatric inpatient aggression. A review of structural and functional assessment approaches. *Aggression and Violent Behavior*, **7**, 477–497.

Dale, C., Thompson, T. & Woods, P. (eds) (2001) *Forensic Mental Health. Issues in Practice*. Baillière Tindall, London.

Dale, C., Gardner, J. & Philogene, S. (2002) Overcoming barriers to change: case of Ashworth Hospital. In: *Managing and Leading Innovations in Health Care* (eds E. Howkins & C. Thornton), pp 220–246. Baillière Tindall, London.

Department of Health (1995) *Building Bridges. A Guide to Arrangements for Interagency Working for the Care and Protection of Severely Mentally Ill People*, p. 88. Department of Health, London.

Department of Health (1999a) *Clinical Governance: Quality in the New NHS*. Department of Health, London.

Department of Health (1999b) *National Confidential Inquiry into Suicide and Homicide by People with Mental Illness*. Department of Health, London.

Department of Health (2002a) *Mental Health Policy Implementation Guide. Dual Diagnosis Good Practice Guide*. Department of Health, London.

Department of Health (2002b) *National Suicide Prevention Strategy for England*. Department of Health, London.

Department of Health (2003) *Mainstreaming Gender and Women's Mental Health. Implementation Guide*. Department of Health, London.

Department of Health (2006) *Self-Assessment Toolkit. From Values to Action: The Chief Nursing Officer's Review of Mental Health Nursing*. Department of Health, London.

Department of Health (2007) *Best Practice in Managing Risk. Principles and Evidence for Best Practice in the Assessment and Management of Risk to Self and Others in Mental Health Services*. Department of Health, London.

Douglas, K.S. & Belfrage, H. (2001) Use of the HCR-20 in violence risk management: implementation and clinical practice. In: *HCR-20 Violence Risk Management Companion Guide* (eds K.S. Douglas, C.D. Webster, S.D. Hart, D. Eaves & J.R.P. Ogloff), pp 41–58. Simon Fraser University, British Columbia.

Doyle, M. (2000) Risk assessment and management. In: *Forensic Mental Health Nursing: Current Approaches* (eds C. Chaloner & M. Coffey), pp 140–170. Blackwell Science, Oxford.

Doyle, M. & Dolan, M. (2002) Violence risk assessment: combining actuarial and clinical information to structure clinical judgements for the formulation and management of risk. *Journal of Psychiatric Mental Health Nursing*, **9**(6), 649–657.

Duggan, C. (1997) Assessing risk in the mentally disordered. *British Journal of Psychiatry*, **170**(32), 1–3.

Easton, J. (2002) *Clinical Leadership and the New NHS*. Paper presented to National Mental Health Nurse Leadership Programme, York, May. Personal Lecture Notes.

Elvins, R. (1989) *Security Information Training Package*. Unpublished manuscript, Rampton Hospital Authority, Retford.

Ewens, A. (2002) The nature and purpose of leadership. In: *Managing and Leading Innovation in Health Care* (eds E. Howkins & C. Thornton), pp 69–90. Baillière Tindall, London.

Forchuk, C. (2001) Evidence-based psychiatric/mental health nursing. *Evidence-Based Mental Health*, **4**, 39–40.

Foy, R., Grimshaw, J. & Eccles, M. (2001) Guidelines and pathways. In: *Clinical Risk Management. Enhancing Patient Safety* (ed. C. Vincent), 2nd edn, pp 283–300. BMJ Books, London.

Grounds, A. (1995) Risk assessment and management in clinical context. In: *Psychiatric Patient Violence: Risk and Response* (ed. J. Crichton), pp 43–59. Duckworth and Company, London.

Gunden, E. & Crissman, S. (1992) Leadership skills for empowerment. *Nursing Administration Quarterly*, **16**(3), 6–10.

Gunn, J. (1993) Dangerousness. In: *Forensic Psychiatry. Clinical, Legal and Ethical Issues* (eds J. Gunn & P. Taylor). Butterworth-Heinemann, London.

Hackett, M., Lilford, R. & Jordan, J. (1999) Clinical governance: culture, leadership, and power – the key to changing attitudes and behaviours in trusts. *International Journal of Health Care Quality Assurance*, **12**(3), 98–104.

Hanson, R.K. (1997) *The Development of a Brief Actuarial Risk Scale for Sexual Offense Recidivism (User Report No. 1997–04)*. Department of the Solicitor General of Canada, Ottawa.

Hanson, R.K. (2004) Sex offender risk assessment. In: *The Essential Handbook of Offender Assessment and Treatment* (ed. C.R. Hollin), pp 31–43. Wiley and Sons, Chichester.

Hare, R.D. (1991) *Manual for the Hare Psychopathy Checklist-Revised*. Multi-Health Systems, Toronto.

Hart, S.D. (2001) Assessing and managing violence risk. In: *HCR-20 Violence Risk Management Companion Guide* (eds K.S. Douglas, C.D. Webster, S.D. Hart, D. Eaves & J.R.P. Ogloff), pp 13–25. Simon Fraser University, British Columbia.

Hart, S.D., Michie, C. & Cooke, D.J. (2007) Precision of actuarial risk assessment procedures. *British Journal of Psychiatry*, **190**(49), 60–65.

Health and Safety Executive (1988) *The Tolerability of Risks from Nuclear Power Stations*. Her Majesty's Stationery Office, London.

Higgins, N., Watts, D., Bindman, J., Slade, M. & Thornicroft, G. (2005) Assessing violence risk in general adult psychiatry. *Psychiatric Bulletin*, **29**(4), 131–133.

Hodgins S. (2004) Offenders with major mental disorders. In: *The Essential Handbook of Offender Assessment and Treatment* (ed. C.R. Hollin), pp 219–230. Wiley and Sons, Chichester.

Hollin, C.R. (1997) Assessing and managing forensic risk: how research findings can contribute to improving practice. *Psychiatric Care*, **4**(5), 212–215.

Hollin, C.R. (ed.) (2004) *The Essential Handbook of Offender Assessment and Treatment*. Wiley and Sons, Chichester.

Holloway, F. (1997) The assessment and management of risk in psychiatry: can we do better? *Psychiatric Bulletin*, **21**(5), 283–285.

Holloway, F. (1998) Risk assessment. *British Journal of Psychiatry*, **173**(12), 540–543.

Howell, J. & Avolio, B. (1993) Transformational leadership, transactional leadership, locus of control, as support for innovation: key predictors of consolidated business unit performance. *Journal of Applied Psychology*, **78**(6), 98–104.

Ireland, J.L. (2004) Compiling forensic risk assessment reports. *Forensic Update*, **77**, 15–22.

Jones, J. & Plowman, C. (2005) Risk assessment: a multidisciplinary approach to estimating harmful behaviour in mentally disordered offenders. In: *Multidisciplinary Working in Forensic Mental Health Care* (eds S. Wix & M. Humphreys), pp 133–150. Elsevier Churchill Livingstone, Oxford.

Kemshall, K. (1999) Risk assessment and risk management: practice and policy implications. *British Journal of Forensic Practice*, **1**(1), 27–36.

Kennedy, H. (2001) Risk assessment is inseparable from risk management. *Psychiatric Bulletin*, **25**(6), 208–211.

Kettles, A.M. (2004) A concept analysis of forensic risk. *Journal of Psychiatric and Mental Health Nursing*, **11**(4), 484–493.

Kettles, A.M., Robinson, D. & Moody, E. (2003) A review of clinical risk and related assessments in forensic psychiatric units. *British Journal of Forensic Practice*, **5**(3), 3–11.

Kohner, N. (1994) *Clinical Supervision in Practice: Work from Nursing Development Units*. Kings Fund Centre, London.

Landrum, N., Howell, J. & Paris, L. (2000) Leadership for strategic change. *Leadership and Organization Development Journal*, **21**(3), 150–156.

Lipsedge, M. (2001) Risk management in psychiatry. In: *Clinical Risk Management. Enhancing Patient Safety* (ed. C. Vincent), 2nd edn, pp 219–240. BMJ Books, London.

MacCall, C. (2003) A review of approaches to forensic risk assessment in Australia and New Zealand. *Psychiatry, Psychology and Law*, **10**(1), 221–226.

Maden, A. (2003) Standardised risk assessment: why all the fuss? *Psychiatric Bulletin*, **27**(6), 201–204.

Maden, A. (2005) Violence risk assessment: the question is not whether but how. *Psychiatric Bulletin*, **29**(4), 121–122.

Malby, B. (1998) Clinical leadership. *Advanced Practice Nursing Quarterly*, **3**(4), 40–43.

Manthorpe, J. & Alaszewski, A. (2000) Service users, informal carers and risks. In: *Managing Risk in Community Practice. Nursing, Risk and Decision Making* (eds A. Alaszewski, H. Alaszewski, S. Ayer & J. Manthorpe), pp 47–70. Baillière Tindall, London.

Marshall, W.L. (2004) Adult sexual offenders against women. In: *The Essential Handbook of Offender Assessment and Treatment* (ed. C.R. Hollin), pp 147–162. Wiley and Sons, Chichester.

Mason, T. (1998) Models of risk assessment in mental health practice: a critical examination. *Mental Health Care*, **1**(12), 405–407.

McGuire, J. (2001) What is problem solving? A review of theory, research and applications. *Criminal Behaviour and Mental Health*, **11**(4), 210–235.

Mercer, D., Mason, T., McKeown, M. & McCann, G. (eds) (2000) *Forensic Mental Health Care: A Case Study Approach*. Churchill Livingstone, London.

Monahan, J. (1981) *The clinical prediction of violent behaviour*. Government Printing Office, Washington, DC.

Monahan, J. (2001) Preface. In: *Rethinking Risk Assessment: The MacArthur Study of Mental Disorder and Violence* (eds J. Monahan, H.J. Steadman, E. Silver, *et al.*), pp v–vii. Oxford University Press, Oxford.

Monahan, J. & Steadman, H.J. (eds) (1994) *Violence and Mental Disorder: Developments In Risk Assessment*. The University of Chicago Press, Chicago.

Monahan, J., Steadman, H.J., Silver, E., *et al.* (eds) (2001) *Rethinking Risk Assessment: The MacArthur Study of Mental Disorder and Violence*. Oxford University Press, Oxford.

Moore, B. (1996) *Risk Assessment: A Practitioner's Guide to Predicting Harmful Behaviour*. Whiting and Birch, London.

Moss, F. & Paice, E. (2001) Training and supervision. In: *Clinical Risk Management: Enhancing Patient Safety* (ed. C. Vincent), 2nd edn, pp 341–354. BMJ Books, London.

Mullen, P. (2002) Serious mental disorder and offending behaviours. In: *Offender Rehabilitation and Treatment: Effective Programmes and Policies to Reduce Re-offending* (ed. J. McGuire), pp 289–305. Wiley and Sons, Chichester.

Munro, E. & Rumgay, J. (2000) Role of risk assessment in reducing homicides by people with mental illness. *British Journal of Psychiatry*, **176**, 116–120.

National Institute for Mental Health in England (2004a) *Mental Health Policy Implementation Guideline. Developing Positive Practice to Support the Safe and Therapeutic Management of Aggression and Violence in Mental Health In-patient Settings*. NIMHE, Leeds.

National Institute for Mental Health in England (2004b) *Emerging Best Practices in Mental Health Recovery*. NIMHE, London.

Neilson, T., Malcolm, M.B., Ledsham, R. & Poole, J. (1996) Does the nursing care plan help in the management of psychiatric risk? *Journal of Advanced Nursing*, **24**(6), 1201–1206.

North East Thames and South East Thames Regional Health Authorities (1994) *Report of the Inquiry into the Care of Christopher Clunis*. Her Majesty's Stationery Office, London.

Novaco, R.W. (1975) *Anger Control: The Development and Evaluation of an Experimental Treatment*. D.C. Heath, Lexington, MA.

Nursing and Midwifery Council (2003) *Preceptorship*. Nursing and Midwifery Council, London.

Ogloff, J.R.P. (2001) Professional, legal and ethical issues in violence risk management. In: *HCR-20 Violence Risk Management Companion Guide* (eds K.S. Douglas, C.D. Webster, S.D. Hart, D. Eaves & J.R.P. Ogloff), pp 59–71. Simon Fraser University, British Columbia.

O'Rourke, M.M., Hammond, S.J. & Davies, E.J. (1997) Risk assessment and risk management: the way forward. *Psychiatric Care*, **4**(3), 104–106.

Perkins, R. (1996) Seen but not heard: can 'user involvement' become more than empty rhetoric? *The Mental Health Review*, **1**(4), 16–20.

Petch, E. (2001) Risk management in UK mental health services: an overvalued idea? *Psychiatric Bulletin*, **25**(6), 203–205.

Pilgrim, D. (1997) Some reflections on 'quality' and 'mental health'. *Journal of Mental Health*, **6**(6), 567–576.

Potts, J. (1995) Risk assessment and management: a Home Office perspective. In: *Psychiatric Patient Violence: Risk and Response* (ed. J. Crichton), pp 35–42. Duckworth and Company, London.

Prins, H. (1999) *Will They Do It Again? Risk Assessment and Management in Criminal Justice and Psychiatry*. Routledge, London.

Prins, H. (2002) Risk assessment: still a risky business. *British Journal of Forensic Practice*, **4**(1), 3–8.

Prins, H. (2005a) The 'crystal ball' of risk assessment. In: *Offenders, Deviants or Patients?* (ed. H. Prins), 3rd edn, pp 261–285. Routledge, Hove.

Prins, H. (2005b) Taking chances: risk assessment and management in a risk obsessed society. *Medicine, Science and the Law*, **45**(2), 93–109.

Quinsey, V.L., Harris, G.T., Rice, M.E. & Cormier, C.A. (1998) *Violent Offenders. Appraising and Managing Risk*. American Psychological Association, Washington, DC.

Rae, M. (2000) *Different Journeys – Same Destination (4th Version)*. Paper presented at the Yorkshire Centre for Forensic Psychiatry, Wakefield, December.

Reed, J. (1997) Risk assessment and clinical risk management: the lessons from recent inquiries. *British Journal of Psychiatry*, **170**(32), 4–7.

Reith, M. (1998) Risk assessment and management: lessons from mental health inquiry reports. *Medicine, Science and the Law*, **38**(3), 221–226.

Robert, C. (2006) Managing risk: from the inside looking out (editorial). *Criminal Behaviour and Mental Health*, **16**(3), 142–145.

Robinson, D. & Collins, M. (1999) Risk assessment: a challenge to nurses and nurse managers. *Mental Health Practice*, **2**(6), 8–13.

Robinson, D. & Kettles, A. (eds) (2000) *Forensic Nursing and Multidisciplinary Care of the Mentally Disordered Offender*. Jessica Kingsley, London.

Robinson, R., Fenwick, J. & Wood, S. (2006) *Report of the Independent Inquiry into the Care and Treatment of John Barrett*. National Health Service, London.

Royal Society (1992) *Risk: Analysis, Perception, Management*. Royal Society, London.

Scott, P. (1977) Assessing dangerousness in criminals. *British Journal of Psychiatry*, **131**, 127–142.

Schultz, J.M. & Videbeck, S.L. (2005) *Lippincott's Manual of Psychiatric Nursing Care Plans*, 7th edn. Lippincott, Williams and Wilkins, Philadelphia.

Secker-Walker, J. & Donaldson, L. (2001) Clinical governance: the context of risk management. In: *Clinical Risk Management: Enhancing Patient Safety* (ed. C. Vincent), 2nd edn, pp 61–73. BMJ Books, London.

Secker-Walker, J. & Taylor-Adams, S. (2001) Clinical incident reporting. In: *Clinical Risk Management: Enhancing Patient Safety* (ed. C. Vincent), 2nd edn, pp 419–438. BMJ Books, London.

Shanley, M.J. & Stevenson, C. (2006) Clinical supervision revisited. *Journal of Nursing Management*, **14**(8), 586–592.

Snowden, P. (1997) Practical aspects of clinical risk assessment and management. *British Journal of Psychiatry*, **170**(32), 32–34.

Spielberger, C.D. (1999) *State-Trait Anger Expression Inventory – 2 (STAXI-2)*. Psychological Assessment Resources Incorporated, Odessa, Florida.

Standing Nursing and Midwifery Advisory Committee (1999) *Practice Guidance: Safe and Supportive Observation of Patients at Risk. Mental Health Nursing: 'Addressing Acute Concerns'*. Department of Health, London.

Steadman, H.J., Monahan, J., Appelbaum, P.S., *et al.* (1994) Designing a new generation of risk assessment research. In: *Violence and Mental Disorder. Developments in Risk Assessment* (eds J. Monahan & H.J. Steadman), pp 297–318. University of Chicago Press, Chicago.

Surgeon General (1999) *Mental Health: A Report of the Surgeon General*. Office of Surgeon General, Washington, DC.

Szmukler, G. (2003) Risk assessment 'numbers' and 'values'. *Psychiatric Bulletin*, **27**(6), 205–207.

Taylor, P. (2001) *Expert Paper: Mental Illness and Serious Harm to Others*. NHS National Programme on Forensic Mental Health Research and Development, Liverpool.

Thompson, D.R. (2000) An exploration of knowledge development in nursing – a personal perspective. *Nursing Times Research*, **5**(5), 391–394.

Tomlin, A., Darnes, K.L. & Badenoch, D.S. (2002) Enabling evidence-based change in health care. *Evidence-Based Mental Health*, **5**, 68–71.

Turner-Crowson, J. & Wallcraft, J. (2002) The recovery vision for mental health services and research: a British perspective. *Psychiatric Rehabilitation Journal*, **25**(3), 245–254.

United Kingdom Central Council for Nursing, Midwifery and Health Visiting (1998) *Guidelines for Mental Health and Learning Disabilities Nursing*. UKCC, London.

Walshe, K. (2001) The development of clinical risk management. In: *Clinical Risk Management: Enhancing Patient Safety* (ed. C. Vincent), 2nd edn, pp 45–60. BMJ Books, London.

Webster, C.D. & Bailes, G. (2004) Assessing violence risk in mentally and personality disordered individuals. In: *The Essential Handbook of Offender Assessment and Treatment* (ed. C.R. Hollin), pp 17–30. Wiley & Sons, Chichester.

Webster, C.D., Douglas, K.S., Eaves, D. & Hart, S.D. (1997) *HCR-20 Assessing Risk for Violence (Version 2)*. Simon Fraser University, British Columbia.

West, A.G. (2001) Current approaches to sex-offender risk assessment: a critical review. *British Journal of Forensic Practice*, **3**(3), 31–41.

Yegdich, T. (1999) Clinical supervision and managerial supervision: some historical and conceptual considerations. *Journal of Advanced Nursing*, **30**(5), 1195–1204.

Chapter 3

The Theory of Risk

Alyson M. Kettles and Phil Woods

Introduction

This chapter focuses on the theoretical aspects of risk assessment and management. The first aim of the chapter is to outline common terminology and define terms clearly. This is important because much confusion surrounds the term 'risk assessment'. For example, many do not realise that the idea of risk is merely another word for 'probability'. The chapter is presented in four parts:

- Part 1 introduces and defines the terms that are in common use.
- Part 2 examines the concepts of the variables involved.
- Part 3 discusses the latest thinking in the field.
- Part 4 introduces the concept of risk management.

Part 1: defining terms

When we talk about risk assessment in mental health services we are interested in the broader probability (risk) of an event or behaviour (outcome). The event or behaviour is the primary area of interest because it is generally associated with a degree of severity. This severity could be in relation to illness symptoms or is sometimes referred to as dangerousness. The impact of this severity is extremely important because it is therefore clearly possible to have a high risk of an outcome with low impact (such as swearing) or conversely low risk of an outcome with high impact (for example, serious violence).

Common terminology/definitions

The original meaning of **risk** (Jacobs 2000; Woods 2001) was as either mathematical or statistical probability related to such pastimes as gambling.

For example, 'taking a gamble' indicated the probability of an event occurring combined with the magnitude of loss or gain that could result from the throw of a die or the turn of a card.

However, in modern usage 'risk' means different things to different groups of people (Doyle 2000; Jacobs 2000), but for both health and social care and for mental health nursing 'risk' is specifically about the safety of staff, patients and carers (Kettles 2004). Risk is about whether or not an event will occur. For example, in gambling a player will take risks and the term 'risk everything on the turn of the dice' refers specifically to when a player can either win or lose an exceptionally large bet on a single throw of the die. This bet can be either money or a business or the player's house or any other life-changing significant item or items. This is also where the term 'losing your shirt' comes from, when in the past players have literally lost everything, including the clothes they stand up in.

Risk is also something the insurance industry invests time and money in. In order to minimise risk, insurers will exclude certain groups of people from being able to hold their policies. For example, many new, young drivers who have fast new sports cars can find it difficult to obtain appropriate insurance, or they have to pay more than other drivers to be able to obtain a policy because they are considered to be a higher risk than other drivers of being involved in crashes and accidents. Other groups include middle-aged men with fast sports cars, and the elderly over the age of 75.

Insurance companies use **probability** to calculate the likely risks and benefits for individuals and groups requiring policies.

Probability (The Editors of Chambers 2006) is the chance or the likelihood of something happening and a **statistical probability** (Miller 1989; Hicks 1990) is the chance or likelihood of an event occurring, often represented on a scale that ranges from 0 to 1: 0 represents no chance of the event occurring, and 1 means that it is certain to occur. When we are expressing the results of research in numerical terms we refer to **probability** as the '*p* **value**' and when reporting positive results we say that in this circumstance we can reject the likelihood that research results were obtained by chance because the *p* value is extremely improbable, i.e. when the *p* value is less than or equal to 0.05. The smaller the *p* value the less likely it is that random errors could explain the results (Siegel and Castellan 1988; Miller 1989; Hicks 1990).

Often when results of risk assessment research are reported this is in terms of the **correlation coefficient**, with researchers frequently highlighting the related *p* value as important, when in fact it is the strength of association found in the correlation that is more of interest. The cautionary note is that when the sample size is large the correlation is likely to be significant yet small in real terms. As a general guide the following has been suggested as specific levels of interest relative to the correlation:

- +0.19 and below can be considered very low;
- +0.20 to +0.39 low;
- +0.40 to +0.69 modest;
- +0.70 to +0.89 high;
- +0.90 to +1.00 very high.

(Cohen and Holliday 1982).

An **event** is any incidence or occurrence and a dictionary definition identifies that an event is 'that which happens' (The Editors of Chambers 2006). So any event or 'outcome' in risk assessment terms is any occurrence of assessment items, such as 'verbal aggression following a trigger event' or participating in 'social activities' which can be measured in some way. According to Morgan (2004, p.18),

> '. . . in the specific field of mental health, "event" frequently refers to behaviours resulting in suicide, self-harm, aggression and violence, and the neglect, abuse and exploitation by self or others'.

Different assessment instruments use different assessment items and different forms of measurement and this will be discussed in more detail in subsequent chapters.

A useful way to consider how events occur is very similar to the way the testing of the predictive ability of many risk assessments takes place by researchers. This is also a good way to evaluate whether outcomes have been successful or not. Two-by-two contingency tables are an excellent way to display these results (see Table 3.1) as it enables correct predictions and error rates to be examined. Two possibilities exist in this design: either the risky event identified did occur or it did not. Typically this is reported as:

- a **true negative** (the patient was predicted to be a risk and the risk event did not occur);
- a **true positive** (the patient was predicted to be a risk and the risk event did occur);
- a **false negative** (the patient was predicted to be not a risk and the risk event did occur);
- a **false positive** (the patient was predicted to be a risk and the risk event did not occur).

Behaviour is about conduct and manners, and the thoughts, cognitions and emotions that are related to the behaviour under assessment. Behaviour is also a physiological response to a stimulus and in the context of risk assessment it is about the ways in which a person responds to staff, other patients, the environment, his or her symptoms, and the various forms of

Table 3.1 An example two-by-two contingency table.

		Outcome	
		Risk event	No risk event
Prediction	Risk event will occur	True positive	False positive
	Risk event will not occur	False negative	True negative

treatment and intervention that he/she may undergo whilst in care in either the hospital or the community. It is also about the recurrence of the behaviour at any given time and about the probability of the behaviour recurring if it is a risky, severe or dangerous behaviour.

The **severity** of behaviour is about the level of intensity during the occurrence and will often be seen referred to as mild, moderate or severe. Especially in relation to risk to others, this severity will be seen termed as 'dangerousness'. **Dangerousness** is when behaviours that cause harm are present or have been known to be present previously. The negative consequences include:

- causing serious physical and psychological harm;
- fear-induction;
- impulsive actions;
- intimidation;
- feeling unsafe;
- peril;
- hazard;
- being at risk;
- insecurity;
- having the power to hurt;
- being manipulative;
- being destructive.

(Kemshall 2001; Woods 2001).

The preferred term for dangerousness in current usage is 'risk'.

Feeling safe or unsafe is a major issue for staff while conducting risk assessments and so **safety** or the state or fact of being safe is important in all aspects of mental health nursing including risk assessment and management.

Security is related to safety and the varying outcomes of risk assessment in mental health nursing (Collins *et al.* 2006). According to Collins (2000), security comes in two forms: physical and relational. Physical security is about the objects (such as doors, fences and locks) and the systems (such as regular procedures and the use of closed circuit television) that are in place to ensure safety. Relational security relates very specifically to risk assessment and management as it entails a depth of knowledge about each individual patient which nurses and patients develop together through the nurse–patient relationship. Relational security can be achieved as an outcome of risk assessment and management through a sound knowledge and understanding of the actual risks posed at any one time, as well as the potential risks and how these might be minimised, and the relevant interventions that are part of appropriate management for each patient.

Having defined these terms, what must now be asked is what are the characteristics of risk? As Doyle (2000, p.142) says: '*Risk means different things to different people*'.

Risk-taking is a daily occurrence in health and social care and clinicians make decisions to take risks with patients as a matter of course. For example, in acute in-patient mental health services patients who have been placed on high-level observation need at some point in their care to have a reduction in the level of observation. At that point in care it becomes a 'risk' to reduce the level of observation, in case the patient is not well enough or has been deceiving the staff, and as a consequence of the reduction the patient harms him- or herself or others. However, this risk is taken because the clinical staff and relevant others, such as the relatives of the patient, decide that, based on all the available evidence and the risk assessments that have been conducted, the patient is ready for the reduction in the level of observations. This has also been termed **positive risk-taking** which:

'. . . is *weighing up the potential benefits and harms of exercising one choice of action over another. This means identifying the potential risks involved, and developing plans and actions that reflect the positive potentials and stated priorities of the service user. It involves using available resources and support to achieve desired outcomes, and to minimise potential harmful outcomes. Positive risk-taking is not negligent ignorance of the potential risks. Nobody, especially users or providers of a specific service or activity, will benefit from allowing risks to play out their course through to disaster'* (Morgan 2004, p.18).

What should be noted here is the use of the terms 'evidence' and 'risk assessments'. **Evidence** is about both the objective and the subjective evidence that is available; for example, reports from other professionals based upon their health assessments, such as dieticians and their use of assessment tools such as the Malnutrition Universal Screening Tool (MUST) (Todorovic *et al.* 2003) as well as specific mental health instruments. The term **risk assessment** relates to both the possible approaches (clinical judgement, structured clinical judgement, the actuarial approach and the normative approach) (MacLean 2000; Kettles 2004) and the numerous and multifaceted instruments (MacLean 2000; Kettles *et al.* 2001, 2003; MacCall 2003; Risk Management Authority 2007) that are available to attempt to quantify what the risk might be at any given time for individuals to commit some level of harm at any given time.

Some of these instruments are about **prediction** of future behaviour and attempt to say that at any given point in the future the person will offend or re-offend. Other instruments are not designed to be predictive and are for use only as a 'snapshot' in time. These tools give a quantification of the existing risk, now, and cannot be used to predict future behaviour.

Many of these risk assessment instruments are considered by their authors to be suitable for use in research rather than in clinical practice. However, some of these instruments have been taken up for use in clinical practice by practitioners because they need a method to be able to say to other people, such as lawyers, that they have based their decisions on some form of **objective** assessment. Objective means that it is not simply your own ideas that matter but that there has been a systematic way of collecting the evidence about the person's state of risk that provides a reasonable way of helping the clinician to come to a decision. This systematic method provides **items** (variables) that have been tested as providing relevant information and which are consistent, valid and reliable in research terms in order to provide the information needed to make decisions about the level of risk a person poses at any given time.

Part 2: variables

Now the concepts of variables and how they contribute to predicting outcome will be examined. This will be achieved by looking at the concepts of **actuarial** (or **static**) variables and **clinical** (or **dynamic**) variables and by providing brief examples from mental health and also broader fields (for example, the insurance industry) to give the reader a firm grounding in the complexities of the subject area.

Risk factors are **variables**, or personal characteristics, situations or environmental conditions that predict the onset, continuity or escalation of risky behaviour. These variables, or personal characteristics, have been shown to have an empirically based (scientifically sound) relationship with the risk in question. These are often considered in terms of type of information, and whether the information is static or dynamic in nature.

Static risk variables are historical in nature and reflect prior life experiences and previous behaviours that are associated with a statistically increased likelihood or probability of the risk behaviour. Static risk variables are considered to be fixed or inert. Whatever degree of risk is implied by these static variables can only change with the introduction of dynamic risk variables. Static risk factors are variables that have been shown to have a relationship with the risk but that are not amenable to clinical intervention. Examples include age, history of violence, offending behaviour and previous convictions. These variables affect the likelihood of a person being risky in the future (for example, re-offending) but cannot be changed by treatment. Static factors, according to Hanson and Bussiere (1998), include such items as:

- prior sexual offences;
- any deviant sexual preference;
- failure to complete treatment;
- any personality disorder;
- anger problems;
- an elevated Psychopathy Check List-Revised (PCL-R) (Hare 1991) score.

A dynamic risk variable must satisfy a number of conditions:

1. It must precede and be associated with risk behaviour.
2. It must be capable of changing.
3. Changing the variable must change or influence or affect the risk behaviour in some way.

Thus, dynamic risk variables must be capable of mitigating (reducing) or exacerbating the risk suggested by static variables. Dynamic risk factors are variables that also have been shown to have a relationship with the risk (using the previous example of re-offending), but these can change as a result of treatment. Examples include:

- individual or environmental aspects;
- symptoms of illness;
- self-harming behaviours;
- drug or alcohol use;
- deviant sexual interest;
- sexual fantasy;
- negative attitudes to women.

Specifically in relation to sex offenders, the National Organisation for the Treatment of Abusers (2007) considers that:

Table 3.2 Some examples of static risk factors, stable dynamic factors and acute dynamic factors.

Static factors (Hanson *et al.* 1995)	Stable dynamic factors (Hanson and Harris 1998)	Acute dynamic factors (Hanson and Harris 1998)
• Antisocial personality disorder	• Sees self as no risk	• Victim access
• Prior criminal offences	• Disengaged	• Overall cooperation
• Anger problems	• Number of positive influences	• Disengaged
• Any personality disorder	• Manipulative	• Anger
• Failure to complete treatment	• Low remorse/victim blaming	• Low remorse/victim blaming
• Sexual interest in children	• Victim access	• Substance misuse
• Negative relationship with mother	• Antisocial lifestyle	• Negative mood
• Early onset of offending	• Number of negative influences	• Sees self as no risk
• Any deviant sexual preference	• Non-attendance/late for treatment	• General hygiene problems
• Victim was a stranger	• Sexual preoccupation	• General social problems
• Offender is less than 23 years old	• Rape attitudes	• Psychiatric symptoms
• Offender is single	• Substance misuse	• Manipulative
• Victim was a male child	• Hygiene problems	• Non-attendance/late for treatment
• Diverse sex crimes	• Unemployment	• Unemployment

'... the identification of dynamic factors that are associated with reduced recidivism holds particular promise in effectively managing sex offenders because the strengthening of these factors can be encouraged through various supervision and treatment strategies'.

Dynamic factors can be further categorised into **stable** and **acute factors** (Hanson and Harris 1998), as shown in Table 3.2. **Stable dynamic factors** are those characteristics that can change over time, but are relatively enduring qualities. For example, these characteristics can include antisocial lifestyle, being manipulative or substance misuse. Hanson and Harris (1998, 2000) suggest that such stable dynamic risk factors also include:

- seeing self as no risk (lack of insight);
- an attitude of sexual entitlement;
- being manipulative;
- sexual preoccupations;
- rape attitudes;
- intimacy deficits;
- negative social influences;
- negative or indifferent attitudes;
- sexual/emotional self-regulation;
- general self-regulation.

Hanson and Harris (1998), however, suggest that **acute dynamic factors** are conditions that can change over short periods of time. Examples include:

- victim access;
- anger;
- low remorse/victim blaming;
- substance abuse;
- the sexual arousal or intoxication that may immediately precede an offence.

The Department of Health (2007, pp.13–14) categorises risk factors based on the work of Kraemer *et al.* (1997) in similar but slightly differing terminology:

'Static factors – those which are unchangeable. For instance, history of violence, offending behaviour. Dynamic factors – those that change over time and make them more amenable to management. For instance, individual or environmental aspects such as substance misuse and social networks. Stable or chronic factors – those dynamic factors that are quite stable and change slowly over time. These could also possibly include the examples given for dynamic factors but of course

*are specific to the individual. Those factors that tend to change rapidly are known as **acute factors** or **triggers** and, as they do change rapidly, their influence on the level of risk may be short-lived.'*

A full and comprehensive risk assessment will bring together all the different risk assessments that the multidisciplinary team will make. These individualised assessments including those with empirically established acute dynamic risk factors, stable dynamic risk factors, static risk factors and situational variables will be used to make decisions about care and treatment.

However, some caution is needed in assessing any risk, given the limited number of characteristics for different types of behaviour that have a known relationship to future risk. Monahan and Steadman (1994) have highlighted that insufficient variables had been used in research up to that time, and that outcome measures had also been poorly defined. However, this is a changing, ever-evolving area of care, and constant updating is required to know the current situation.

Causes of offending behaviour and inference

Can we say that risk variables cause offending behaviour? We can only say yes when it has been demonstrated, empirically, that changing the risk variable results in changes in the onset or continuity of offending or recidivism. Otherwise, we must assume that risk variables are simply correlated (a relationship that is non-causal) with offending behaviour. In research terms we tend to talk about causation and what we can infer (**inference**) from the statistics we use. Some statistics are descriptive and from these we cannot infer that the results mean there is a causal relationship between two or more variables. Inferential statistics do more than descriptive statistics because they provide us with what can be inferred as causal relationships between variables.

Actuarial risk assessment scales

The work done by actuaries, who are people trained to calculate risks using statistics, commonly for insurance companies, law firms, large companies or bookmakers, is said to be **actuarial**. Actuarial scales are constructed and developed using statistical analysis of groups of people with known outcomes (for example, men who have been convicted of a particular sex offence and men who apparently have not re-offended sexually). This form of analysis tells us which items do the best job of differentiating between those who re-offended and those who seemingly did not re-offend if we use our sexual offending example. Since some variables do a better job than others, these analyses can also tell us how much each variable should be weighted, if at all. These variables are then combined to form a risk assessment scale. This scale is then tested to see how well it works at making a prediction about those who, again if we use our sexual offending example, are likely to re-offend. These types of study provide evidence and support for the predictive validity of the scale.

The risk assessment scale is then used on different samples to see how well it works. This is known as cross-validation. When a scale has been used on many differing samples, including those that are able to provide normative scores, the scale score can then be used as an estimate of the probability that the individual will or will not have the risk within a specified time. For example, an individual male offender with a particular score on a particular risk assessment scale might have a 35% probability of re-offending within 5 years; or a particular young woman with borderline personality disorder who is displaying certain behaviours is more at risk from self-harm.

Actuarial scales often appear to work better when variables are weighted. Item weighting considers that some variables are more important than others when it comes to predicting outcome. Item weighting is done with a statistical method known as multiple linear regression analysis. The result is a 'weighted linear prediction'. Item weighting, however, is not mandatory in risk assessment development. Some argue that simple unit item weighting, where each variable is weighted equally, is just as effective. The Psychopathy Check List-Revised (PCL-R) (Hare 1991), for instance, is a simple unit item weighting. All items are scored 0, 1 or 2.

Item weighting is a scientific question. In order to conduct item weighting, large samples are required to determine the item weights, and the resulting judgments must be made empirically. Some risk assessment scales use 'clinically derived' weightings where clinicians decided the relative importance of each item and weighted each item according to their own clinical judgment. This is not an acceptable situation. Without sufficient data to suggest otherwise, items should have equal weights.

Historically, there has been a 'clinical versus actuarial' debate, where people have argued that only actuarial scales gave an accurate risk assessment and that these should be used clinically as opposed to the clinical scales that tried to give an overall picture of an individual's situation. However, in many respects this debate has been superseded by the advent of structured clinical judgement which uses actuarial assessments as the basis for an overall picture of the patient which enables decision making based on both types of assessment. This development is useful for clinicians and researchers alike as it takes risk assessment to new and more appropriate levels, such as comparison of different actuarial assessments in clinical practice and also the development of normative scales, such as the BEST-Index

(Ross *et al*. 2007; Woods 2008), for use over time rather than just the traditional 'snapshot in time' approach.

Can the scores of risk scales be 'adjusted'?

The question of whether or not a researcher or a clinician should 'adjust' the numerical score from an actuarial scale based upon knowledge of important information that the scale does not take into account or does not emphasise is a matter of some controversy. Those who recommend adjustment do so because the clinician or researcher may be privy to potentially critical information that could affect risk but which is not addressed (or not adequately addressed) by the scale being used in the clinical area at that time. Examples might include being very depressed or very angry after being kicked out of the house, having a partner or girl-/boyfriend suddenly end a relationship, or having a very important person die (or be killed). When risk assessment is close in time to these types of acute events, it is obviously important to take note of them and include them in the overall picture of risk.

It is not recommended, however, that the score of any empirically validated risk assessment scale ever be changed without recourse to revalidation of the scale. The most important reason is that it is very difficult, if not impossible, to provide adequate ground rules for ensuring uniform adjustment in the field. How much a score is adjusted and under what circumstances the adjustment is made is left up to the individual clinician or researcher, introducing both error and unreliability. Changing the score of a risk assessment scale based on such 'new' information is equivalent to changing the T-score on the Minnesota Multiphasic Personality Inventory (MMPI) scale after recognising that the client's score on that scale does not reflect this 'new' information. It would clearly be highly unethical to change T-scores on standardised tests. It is, in the authors' estimation, equally unethical to change the scores on validated risk assessment scales.

So, how do we take into account information that is clearly important in assessing risk? We recommend that critical, risk-relevant information be incorporated into a comprehensive multidisciplinary assessment of risk. Rather than attempting to adjust the numerical score of the scale, we consider that it is only proper, and we recommend, that such information be used to 'adjust' the conclusions of the overall risk assessment. All information obtained is presented, along with the score that most accurately reflects the scale. The conclusions might, if appropriate, include the following:

> 'Although the "risk assessment scale" score is relatively low, there are obvious aggravating issues in the individual's life that may increase his risk and these include . . .'.

In effect what is being said is that actuarial factors should serve as an anchor for more dynamic clinical risk assessment. This has been termed third generation research or **structured clinical judgement** (Doyle and Dolan 2002).

What, if anything, can you do to improve your reliability when scoring on validated scales?

Presuming that the items on the scale you are using are clearly stated and that the criteria for scoring the items are also clearly stated, the single most important factor contributing to unreliability is the ambiguity of the information being used to score the items. How clear or how ambiguous the information is can vary enormously from one individual to another. There are no infallible methods for dealing with ambiguous information.

To improve reliability as much as possible, we strongly recommend that clinicians and researchers use as many sources of information as possible when scoring the scale variables and items. In addition, where possible, we recommend that the scale be scored by two independent clinicians who then compare and discuss their scores to minimise the likelihood of error. The agreed upon scores should then be used. When the information from all the available sources is limited, unclear or incomplete, items should be scored 'conservatively' (in the direction of lower risk), and it should be noted here that the resulting score may underestimate the risk.

Clinicians in all disciplines who are using specific scales should, of course, study the Manual prepared for that scale. Lastly, it is always helpful to complete training, and the associated training on case examples, before using the scale on a 'real' individual. The importance of adequate training on practice cases cannot be overstated.

Part 3: latest thinking

This part discusses the latest thinking in risk assessment and management (for example, decision tree analysis) and provides a brief overview of other terminology that the reader may come across (for example, Receiver Operating Characteristic (ROC) analysis). The concept of 'social risk' and how it relates to the risk and dangerousness debate are also discussed.

Risk assessment is a growing field that has moved on considerably from its humble beginnings where clinicians attempted to predict the level of danger that a particular patient represented to the community when freed from state care (Monahan and Steadman 1994). Major changes have taken place, and are continuing to take place. The most recent changes include the setting up of Risk Management Authorities (Risk Management Authority

2007) and the changes to the approaches taken to the assessment of risk to others (MacLean 2000). There are also many risk assessment and management initiatives underway in England and Wales in many aspects of mental health. Although the dedicated programme through the National Institute for Mental Health in England (NIHME) has now closed, risk is clearly on the agenda, with a recent Department of Health (2007) publication entitled *Best Practice in Managing Risk: Principles and Evidence for Best Practice in the Assessment and Management of Risk to Self and Others in Mental Health Services*.

Previously, the situation existed where patients would often find themselves in a situation of either under-restriction or over-restriction and subjected to non-systematic clinical judgement and the 'gut instinct' of the assessing clinician (usually a single individual). Whereas now the situation is that patients, especially within a secure environment, will be subject to the emerging new political context (MacLean 2000; Criminal Justice (Scotland) Act 2003; Mental Health (Care and Treatment) (Scotland) Act 2003) that emphasises the 'least restrictive environment' (sometimes!) in both the criminal justice system and the mental health system. There also exists a vast literature on risk prediction, risk assessment and risk management, which clinicians and researchers did not have access to 20 years ago.

In the international arena the picture is a little different as there is still indeterminate sentencing for forensic patients (in the USA, Canada, Australia and New Zealand), hospital commitment (the USA, England and Wales – Dangerous and Severe Personality Disorder (DSPD), the Netherlands – Ter Beschikking Stelling (TBS) and Germany) and sexually violent predator laws, such as those in the USA and many countries of the world. There is also major service development taking place.

In Scotland the establishment of the Risk Management Authority (RMA) represents a major development, with its primary aim and function being to ensure the effective assessment and management of risk in violent and sexual offenders, for life. This has meant changes to the law to enable this function to happen (www.rmascotland.gov.uk/).

Orders for lifelong restriction are now being given for serious offences which are subject to an order for life if the individual is found to be high risk by accredited RMA Assessors. At the moment the RMA uses and approves the use of what can be termed 'standard' risk assessment instruments (http://www.rmascotland.gov.uk/rmapublications.aspx), such as the Historical Clinical Risk (HCR-20) and the Violence Risk Appraisal Guide (VRAG), in conjunction with the structured clinical judgement approach (MacLean 2000; Kettles 2004). These standard risk assessments are listed in the RMA's *Risk Assessment Tools Evaluation Directory* (2007) and provide some specific instruments and some for general use. However, it is not a comprehensive document and does not prevent raters from using tools with little or no validation. It also includes the PCL-R despite this instrument not being a risk assessment tool. So there does need to be some caution about its use.

As has been mentioned, the area of risk assessment is a growing, evolving, ever-changing field. This is also true of the risk assessment instruments and methods themselves. Not only do the 'standard' risk assessment instruments exist but also some of the newer forms of risk assessment that are currently being extended for use in the fields of mental health care and forensic mental healthcare can easily be found on websites.

For example, **Decision Tree Analysis** (Quinlan 1987) is used to choose the best course of action when you face uncertainty. In many cases a clinician faces an unknown, such as whether or not a patient with a history of violent offences will re-offend after discharge, or if a patient with schizophrenia will disengage from the service. This unknown appears to make it impossible to choose the appropriate option with any certainty. Although the clinician does not know what the likely outcome will be, he or she does generally have knowledge about the possible outcomes and how those outcomes are likely to occur. It is this information that can be used to select the option that is most acceptable and/or likely to produce the best results.

In using decision trees, you need to begin by writing down the decision that you need to make on the left side of a sheet of paper. You may require a large sheet depending on the length of the process. This decision is represented by a small square. Squares represent decisions, while circles represent uncertain outcomes. Write the decision above the square. From the square, draw lines, going right, for each possible solution you can think of. Make sure that the lines are as far apart as possible as you will need space to add material or to put down your thoughts later. At the end of each line, stop and consider what these results mean. If you have reached another decision then draw a square at the end of the line. If it is difficult to know the outcome, then draw a circle. Write in the decisions above the squares and the uncertain outcomes above the circles. If you have completed a solution at the end of a line then leave it with no notation, i.e. just leave it blank. Starting from the lines that now have squares on the end, draw out more lines representing the possible options that you could choose to take. Note what each means along the line. From the circles draw lines that represent possible outcomes, noting the meaning. Keep going until you have drawn as many possible solutions, decisions and outcomes as you can. An example is shown in Figure 3.1.

The calculated values that you are going to assign to each decision or outcome should be added to the decision tree, and an example is shown in Figure 3.2. The values that are calculated for each risk decision tree are relevant to the type of risk under scrutiny. So for a company that is worried about spending money on the development of a new product, financial

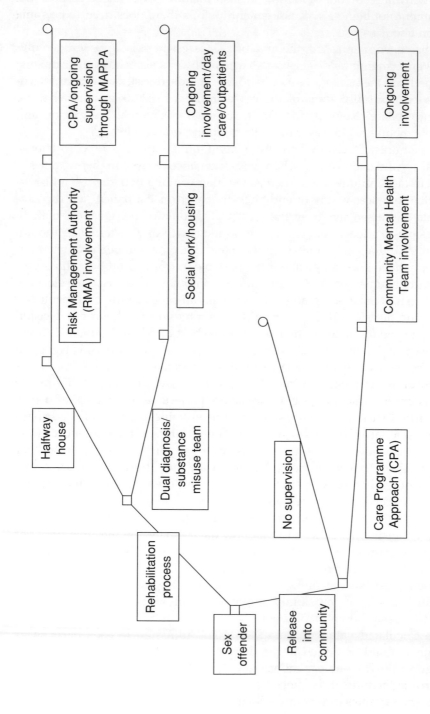

Figure 3.1 An example of a decision tree.

calculations will be made to help decide whether or not the risk is likely to be worth the outlay. In mental health it is more likely that the calculations will be from the various assessments made, including psychological assessment. These assessments will have values assigned, and these may include actuarial assessments with p values which can be used to make decisions.

In Figure 3.2 it can be seen that the sexual offender with a history of violence has a high probability in the poor outcome for being released back into the community with no supervision. This individual also has a high probability of a good outcome for the rehabilitation process, with a halfway house, Risk Management Authority and CPA involvement in care, with ongoing supervision through Multi-Agency Public Protection Arrangements (MAPPA). All the other decisions and outcomes have varying levels of probability which are lower than in these two possible outcomes.

Decision trees provide effective ways of making decisions because they provide:

1. A clear layout of the problem so that each possibility can be challenged and considered.
2. A full analysis of the potential consequences of each decision.
3. A framework by which each potential outcome can be quantified and the probabilities of achieving those outcomes.
4. An opportunity to make the best possible decisions based on existing information and, where relevant, best guesses.

This kind of analysis should only be used as one part of an overall assessment in a decision-making process by the team involved in care. Currently researchers are using this classification tree approach to help develop more useful risk assessment tools and approaches and results appear encouraging (Steadman *et al.* 2000).

Another possible method of determining the extent of risk is **Receiver Operating Characteristics (ROC) analysis** (Rice and Harris 1995; Swets 1996; Harris and Rice 2003; Pepe 2003). ROC analysis is a graphical representation of the trade-off between the false negative and false positive rates for every possible cut-off point on a scale. Put another way (where TP is true positive, FP is false positive, TN is true negative and FN is false negative), it is the trade-off between the sensitivity of an instrument (TP/(TP + FN)) or how often a prediction of the risk occurring is correct, and the specificity (TN/(TN + FP)) or how often a prediction that the risk will not occur is correct. The basic idea of ROC analysis is the mapping of instances into a certain class or group and it can be used, for example, as a method to differentiate between the violent and the non-violent patient. This involves calculating sensitivity and specificity of the test at every possible cut-off and plotting the values of sensitivity against 1-specificity to form a curve. Many computer programs are available to assist in this task.

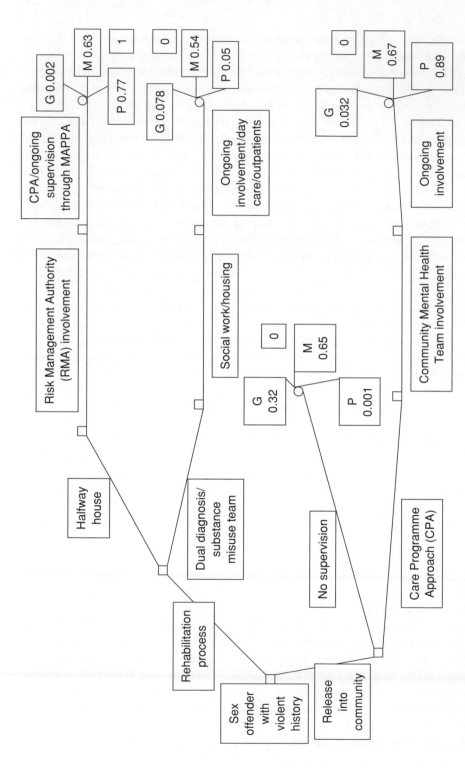

Figure 3.2 An example of a decision tree with values. G = good; M = moderate; P = poor.

A real example of this can be found in the validation studies of the Brøset Violence Checklist (BVC) where it was used as a further method of examining the potential utility of the BVC in the differentiation between the non-violent patient and the violent patient (Almvik *et al.* 2007). The Area Under the Curve (AUC) represents elevation and reflects the BVC's efficiency across its entire range of scores. This is interpreted as the possibility that a randomly selected violent individual will have a higher score than a randomly selected non-violent individual. An AUC of 0.5 is indicative of chance level predictive accuracy, while less than 0.5 is below chance accuracy and greater than 0.5 indicates above chance accuracy. It is the elevation and the shape of the ROC curve that is of most interest and tells you something about the prediction. For example, a curve that has a prominent elbow reaching close to the top left chart corner represents a cut-off score that maximises overall predictive accuracy (specificity 100% and sensitivity 100%).

An example of a ROC analysis from some of the second author's (P.W.) unpublished research work is shown in Figure 3.3, with the AUC 0.835 (SE = 0.04) and a 95% confidence interval (CI) of 0.75–0.92. This represents a highly significant improvement over chance, with probability $p < 0.001$. So ROC analysis can be used to useful effect in mental health and in forensic mental health when assessing the validity of risk assessment instruments and working with prediction.

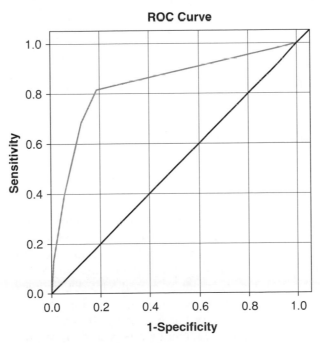

Figure 3.3   An example of a receiver operating characteristic (ROC) curve.

Part 4: the concept of risk management

In this part the concept of risk management and its relationship to the risk assessment process is introduced. Whilst many readers may not be required to go into great depth in these areas it is important that these theoretical foundations are laid and can be related to in the rest of the book.

Risk assessment is not a single entity. It goes hand in hand with a management process that enables the person on the receiving end of the process to have confidence in the staff that there will be appropriate, safe and caring intervention to enable the person to participate in his or her care and to move towards an individual recovery. Indeed, the Department of Health (2007, p.7) highlights that *'risk management is a core component of mental healthcare and the Care Programme Approach'*. Recovery is different for every person and should not always be taken to mean that a 'cure' will be effected. Risk management is the process or intervention through which identified risks are reduced or alleviated (Woods 2008). Put another way, it is vitally important that once a risk assessment has occurred that a risk management plan focuses on the likelihood of the probability or outcome occurring (Woods 2001). Risk management may become a lifelong process for a particular individual or it may be a single 'one-off' event, depending on the circumstances, diagnosis and severity.

Doyle (1999, p.41) defined risk management as:

'. . . the systematic, organised effort to eliminate or reduce the likelihood of misfortune, harm, damage or loss'.

Doyle (2000) further identifies a risk management cycle with several stages including:

- identification and screening;
- assessment;
- control and management;
- monitoring and review.

Doyle considers that this type of cycle is usually implicit to the provision of good quality healthcare and that it should be linked to systematic working in mental healthcare, examples of which include the Care Programme Approach (CPA) and the Risk Management Authority (RMA). Vinestock (1996) describes risk management as a method of balancing probable consequences of decisions which assists in formalising the decision-making process in relation to the risk of harm to self or others.

Usually there is a risk management strategy in each healthcare organisation which determines the ways in which each individual member of staff and each ward, clinical area and department deals with risk assessment and everyday management as a part of the duty of care. Woods (2001) suggests that a strategy should include organisational, cultural, clinical, employee, environmental and incident reporting issues.

Risk management is about reduction of risk and the use of measures that are likely to minimise risk. These measures will be included as either part of the overall strategy or part of the individual's care plan. For example, observation and engagement of the patient is a part of care but it is also a part of policy, guidelines and strategy (Clinical Resource and Audit Group 2002). The Department of Health (2007, p.14) states:

'. . . the aim of risk management is first to assess the likelihood of risk events and then to work with the service user to identify ways of reducing the likelihood of them occurring. Risk management should be based on a plan to reduce the risk of harm occurring and increase the potential for a positive outcome'.

The Department of Health has identified a number of best practice points for effective risk management and these can be found in Box 3.1.

Managing risk is about the response to the risk reflecting the nature of the risk and this should be managed on several levels simultaneously. Primarily the manager of risk should, where possible, prevent harm occurring and this represents direct patient care with proactive measures, such as observation, security and restrictions on access to the means for violence.

Secondary measures include the actions taken after an incident has occurred and include reporting systems, data collection and feedback, complaints and the involvement of the police and legal systems of the country where the incident took place. For example, in Scotland if a completed suicide has occurred in a psychiatric hospital the Procurator Fiscal (Coroner) may direct that a Fatal Accident Inquiry (FAI) is required to ascertain the circumstances surrounding the event. Nursing staff are required to give evidence at an FAI and must produce the evidence of their risk assessments and the associated care planning, including the evidence related to observation level and how that intervention was conducted.

Risk management therefore is not only a policy requirement but also a legal requirement which involves all nursing staff and involves those nursing staff in unidisciplinary and multidisciplinary risk assessment activities. These activities include:

- screening;
- conducting nursing and multidisciplinary risk assessments;
- reviewing those assessments;
- meeting with the patient and with staff about progress.

Box 3.1   Best practice points for effective risk management (Department of Health 2007, pp. 5–6).

1. Best practice involves making decisions based on knowledge of the research evidence, knowledge of the individual service user and his/her social context, knowledge of the service user's own experience, and clinical judgement.
2. Positive risk management as part of a carefully constructed plan is a required competence for all mental health practitioners.
3. Risk management should be conducted in a spirit of collaboration and based on a relationship between the service user and his/her carers that is as trusting as possible.
4. Risk management must be built on a recognition of the service user's strengths and should emphasise recovery.
5. Risk management requires an organisational strategy as well as efforts by the individual practitioner.
6. Risk management involves developing flexible strategies aimed at preventing any negative event from occurring or, if this is not possible, minimising the harm caused.
7. Risk management should take into account that risk can be both general and specific, and that good management can reduce and prevent harm.
8. Knowledge and understanding of mental health legislation is an important component of risk management.
9. The risk management plan should include a summary of all risks identified, formulations of the situations in which identified risks may occur, and actions to be taken by practitioners and the service user in response to crisis.
10. Where suitable tools are available, risk management should be based on assessment using the structured clinical judgement approach.
11. Risk assessment is integral to deciding on the most appropriate level of risk management and the right kind of intervention for a service user.
12. All staff involved in risk management must be capable of demonstrating sensitivity and competence in relation to diversity in race, faith, age, gender, disability and sexual orientation.
13. Risk management must always be based on awareness of the capacity for the service user's risk level to change over time, and a recognition that each service user requires a consistent and individualised approach.
14. Risk management plans should be developed by multidisciplinary and multi-agency teams operating in an open, democratic and transparent culture that embraces reflective practice.
15. All staff involved in risk management should receive relevant training, which should be updated at least every 3 years.
16. A risk management plan is only as good as the time and effort put into communicating its findings to others.

Therapeutic activity and documentation are also a part of the overall care and planning process related to risk assessment, as is management of all of this.

There are some good chapters about risk management (Doyle 2000; Woods 2001; Doyle and Duffy 2006) and the reader is directed to these for further reading.

Risk management is about formalising the decision-making process that results from the risk assessment. The decisions that are made focus on the likely outcome and the outcome that is being aimed for in any individual's case. So, for example, the management plan that is designed for a person who has committed arson and who finds him- or herself in secure care may find that the plan initially restricts access to fire-making equipment, even if he/she smokes cigarettes. The individual will have to ask staff for access to cigarettes and a lighter or matches and will then have to smoke the cigarette under supervision. The plan will likely have various therapeutic activities related to safety, the person's psychological need to set fires, emotional control and attitude, anger management and specific daily activities such as cooking. The plan will also detail which risk and other assessments will be conducted, by whom and when, and the review dates for these over a specified period of time. The management plan will also state what targets the individual is expected to achieve and what to do when they are achieved, as well as what will happen if the target(s) are not achieved, such as review the timescale, reduce the targets, increase input, involve other professionals for specific reasons or other action.

The Department of Health (2007, p.8) proposes that positive risk management is a fundamental of practice where:

> '. . . decisions about risk management involve improving the service user's quality of life and plans for recovery, while remaining aware of the safety needs of the service user, their carer and the public. . . . Overdefensive practice is bad practice. Avoiding all possible risks is not good for the service user or society in the long term, and can be counterproductive, creating more problems than it solves'.

This is an extremely important point and, taken alongside positive risk taking, means that mental health nurses cannot be avoiding risks but need to find ways to work whilst also considering issues of safety. In reality this perhaps means that our patients need to be allowed to make mistakes at times and consequently suffer the consequences if they are to grow and learn from the risks they pose. For those wanting to read more around risk management the Department of Health (2007) is an extremely good starting point.

Conclusion

Risk assessment and risk management go hand-in-hand and cannot be separated or conducted in isolation from each other. In any mental health setting there is a need for nursing staff to be able to conduct risk assessment(s) and then to be able to use appropriate risk management for the benefit of the patient and all those around them, as a part of rigorous, therapeutic caring directed towards recovery. This chapter has outlined some of the words and definitions that nurses need to know and to use in practice. It has also introduced some of the basic concepts associated with risk assessment and management, and discussed a few of the newer methods coming into use in mental practice. Finally, this chapter has ended with a brief discussion of some of the issues related to risk management.

References

Almvik, R., Woods, P. & Rasmussen, K. (2007) Assessing risk for imminent violence in the elderly: the Brøset Violence Checklist. *International Journal of Geriatric Psychiatry,* **22**(9), 862–867.

Clinical Resource and Audit Group (2002) *Engaging People: A Good Practice Statement.* Clinical Resource and Audit Group, Scottish Executive, Edinburgh.

Cohen, L. & Holliday, M. (1982) *Statistics for Social Scientists: An Introductory Text with Computer Programs in Basic.* Harper and Row, London.

Collins, M. (2000) The practitioner new to the role of forensic psychiatric nurse in the UK. In: *Forensic Nursing and Multidisciplinary Care of the Mentally Disordered Offender* (eds D.K. Robinson & A.M. Kettles), pp. 39–50. Jessica Kingsley, London.

Collins, M., Davies, S. & Ashwell, C. (2006) The assessment of security need. In: *Forensic Mental Health Nursing: Interventions with People with 'Personality Disorder'* (ed. The National Forensic Nurses' Research and Development Group). Quay Books, MA Healthcare, London.

Department of Health (2007) *Best Practice in Managing Risk: Principles and Evidence for Best Practice in the Assessment and Management of Risk to Self and Others in Mental Health Services.* Department of Health, London.

Doyle, M. (1999) Organizational responses to crisis and risk: issues and implications for mental health nurses. In: *Managing Crisis and Risk in Mental Health Nursing* (ed. T. Ryan), pp. 40–56. Stanley Thornes, Cheltenham.

Doyle, M. (2000) Risk assessment and management. In: *Forensic Mental Health Nursing: Current Approaches* (eds C. Chaloner & M. Coffey), pp. 140–170. Blackwell Science, Oxford.

Doyle, M. & Dolan, M. (2002) Violence risk assessment: combining actuarial and clinical information to structure clinical judgments for the formulation and management of risk. *Journal of Psychiatric and Mental Health Nursing*, **9**, 649–657.

Doyle, M. & Duffy, D. (2006) Assessing and managing risk to self and others. In: *Forensic Mental Health Nursing: Interventions with People with 'Personality Disorder'* (ed. The National Forensic Nurses' Research and Development Group), pp. 135–150. Quay Books, MA Healthcare, London.

Hanson, R.K. & Bussiere, M.T. (1998) Predicting relapse: a meta-analysis of sexual offender recidivism. *Journal of Consulting and Clinical Psychology*, **66**(2), 348–362.

Hanson, R.K. & Harris, A. (1998) *Dynamic Predictors of Sexual Recidivism*. Corrections Research Ottawa, Department of the Solicitor General, Canada. Available at www.sgc.gc.ca/epub/corr/el99801b/el99801b.htm (accessed 18 October 2007).

Hanson, R.K. & Harris, A. (2000) Where should we intervene? Dynamic predictors of sexual offence recidivism. *Criminal Justice and Behavior*, **27**(1), 6–35.

Hanson, R.K., Scott, H. & Steffy, R.A. (1995) A comparison of child molesters and nonsexual criminals: risk predictors and long-term recidivism. *Journal of Research in Crime and Delinquency*, **32**(3), 325–337.

Hare, R.D. (1991) *The Hare Psychopathy Checklist-Revised*. Multi-Health Systems, Toronto.

Harris, A. & Rice, M. (2003) Actuarial assessment of risk among sex offenders. *Annual New York Academy of Science*, **989**, 198–210.

Hicks, C. (1990) *Research and Statistics: A Practical Introduction for Nurses*. Prentice-Hall, Hemel Hempstead.

Jacobs, L. (2000) An analysis of the concept of risk. *Cancer Nursing*, **23**, 12–19.

Kemshall, H. (2001) *Risk Assessment and Management of Known Sexual and Violent Offenders: A Review of Current Issues*. RDSD Police Research Series Paper 140. Home Office, London.

Kettles, A.M. (2004) A concept analysis of forensic risk. *Journal of Psychiatric and Mental Health Nursing*, **11**(4), 484–493.

Kettles, A.M., Robinson, D.K. & Moody, E. (2001) Brief report: a review of clinical risk and related assessments in forensic psychiatric units. *Journal of Psychiatric and Mental Health Nursing*, **8**, 281–283.

Kettles, A.M., Robinson, D.K. & Moody, E. (2003) A review of clinical risk and related assessments in forensic psychiatric units. *British Journal of Forensic Practice*, **5**, 3–12.

Kraemer, H., Kazdin, A., Offord, D., Kessler, R., Jensen, P. & Kupfer, D. (1997) Coming to terms with the terms of risk. *Archives of General Psychiatry*, **54**(4), 337–343.

MacCall, C. (2003) A review of approaches to forensic risk assessment in Australia and New Zealand. *Psychiatry, Psychology and Law*, **10**, 221–226.

MacLean, Lord (Chairman) (2000) *Report of the Committee on Serious Violent and Sexual Offenders. Executive Summary*. Scottish Executive, Edinburgh.

Miller, S. (1989) *Experimental Design and Statistics*, 2nd edn. Routledge, London.

Monahan, J. & Steadman, H.J. (1994) Towards a rejuvenation of risk assessment research. In: *Violence and Mental Disorder: Developments in Risk Assessment* (eds J. Monahan & H.J. Steadman). University of Chicago Press, Chicago.

Morgan, S. (2004) Positive risk-taking: an idea whose time has come. *Health Care Risk Report*, October, 18–19.

National Organisation for the Treatment of Abusers (2007) *Frequently Asked Questions – Section C. Risk Assessment*. Available at http://www.nota.co.uk/index.php?id=faqrisk_c (accessed 21 February 2008).

Pepe, M.S. (2003) *The Statistical Evaluation of Medical Tests for Classification and Prediction*. Oxford University Press, Oxford.

Quinlan, J.R. (1987) Simplifying decision trees. *International Journal of Man–Machine Studies*, **27**, 221–234.

Rice, M.E. & Harris, G.T. (1995) Violent recidivism – assessing predictive validity. *Journal of Consulting and Clinical Psychology*, **6**(5), 737–748.

Risk Management Authority (2007) *Risk Assessment Tools Evaluation Directory (RATED Version 2)*. Risk Management Authority, Paisley. Available at http://www.rmascotland.gov.uk/rmapublications.aspx (accessed 17 October 2007).

Ross, T., Woods, P., Reed, V., *et al.* (2007) Selecting and monitoring living skills in forensic mental health care: cross-border validation of the BEST-Index. *International Journal of Mental Health*, **36**(4), 3–17.

Siegel, S. & Castellan, N.J. (1988) *Nonparametric Statistics for the Behavioural Sciences*, 2nd edn. McGraw-Hill, New York.

Steadman, H.J., Silver, E., Monahan, J., *et al.* (2000) A classification tree approach to the development of actuarial risk assessment tools. *Law and Human Behavior*, **24**(1), 83–100.

Swets, J.A. (1996) *Signal detection theory and ROC analysis in psychology and diagnostics: collected papers*. Lawrence Erlbaum Associates, Philadelphia.

The Editors of Chambers (2006) *The Chambers Dictionary*, 10th edn. Chambers Harrap, London.

Todorovic, V., Russell, C., Stratton, R., Ward, J. & Elia, M. (2003) *The 'MUST' Explanatory Booklet: A Guide to the 'Malnutrition Universal Screening Tool' (MUST) for Adults*. Malnutrition Advisory Group (MAG) Standing Committee of the British Association for Parenteral and Enteral Nutrition (BAPEN), Redditch.

Vinestock, M. (1996) Risk assessment: 'a word to the wise'? *Advances in Psychiatric Treatment*, **2**, 3–10.

Woods, P. (2001) Risk assessment and management. In: *Forensic Mental Health Care: Issues in Practice* (eds C. Dale, T. Thompson & P. Woods), pp. 85–98. Baillière Tindall/Royal College of Nursing, Edinburgh.

Woods, P. (2008) The forensic mental health nurse's role in risk assessment, measurement and management. In: *Forensic Nursing: Roles, Capabilities and Competencies* (National Forensic Nurses' Research and Development Group, eds A. Kettles, P. Woods & R. Byrt), Chapter 10. Quay Books, London.

Chapter 4

Instrumentation

Phil Woods and Alyson M. Kettles

Introduction

Throughout the research literature, the array of websites that are developing, conference presentations and local service reports, one does not have to look far to find many instruments that are available for assessing all domains of risk that mental health nurses will come across in their everyday practice. Some of these instruments have been developed, or are currently developing, around reliable and valid research studies, whilst others have developed around less formal ways and consequently raise questions about how useful they are. This chapter introduces some of the many instruments and processes that are available to assess and manage risk. It includes issues of appropriate use, including issues of licensing, publisher agreements and appropriate training. The chapter also focuses on the detailed research required to develop such instruments.

Developing instruments for risk assessment

It is the chapter authors' view that instruments used to assess and manage risk by mental health nurses should have been developed via rigorous research, considering the impact these assessments have on health and related behaviours; and any poorly contrived instruments or the development of such instruments without the appropriate strategies and resources in place should be discouraged. For instance, would you drive a car that was not reliable? Therefore should it not be similarly important for assessments of risk you use to be equally reliable for their purpose?

As will emerge through this chapter, many reliable and valid instruments already exist to assess most aspects of risk, so what is the point in 're-inventing the wheel' when it is so much easier to gain access to those that have gone through, or are currently undergoing, the rigorous process of research and development.

Reliability and validity

The development of any assessment instrument involves two fundamental components: reliability and validity. A seminal quote sums the issues up:

> *'If one does not know the reliability and validity of one's data little faith can be put in the results obtained and conclusions drawn from the results'* (Kerlinger 1973, p.442).

Robson (1993, p.66) indicates that this is about establishing 'trustworthiness' or that findings from your enquires are noteworthy. Furthermore, reliability and validity cannot exist in isolation from each other (Robson 1993, p.67; Bryman and Cramer 1997, p.62).

Bech (1994, p.293) puts forward a model for evaluation: first, the construct validity of a scale; second, the external validity; and third, the inter-rater reliability. This model encompasses:

- the representativeness of the items;
- the extent to which items contribute towards the scale;
- the correspondence to other empirical variables or the prediction of behaviour;
- the 'communicative aspect of the scale'.

To be **reliable** something needs to be relied on; to be of sound and consistent character or quality (Oxford University Press 1995). In research terms reliability has been defined as:

- dependability (Kerlinger 1973);
- stability (Kerlinger 1973);
- consistency (Kerlinger 1973);
- predictability (Kerlinger 1973);
- accuracy (Kerlinger 1973);
- consistency, external and internal (Bryman and Cramer 1997, p.63);
- how consistently an empirical scale measures a given phenomenon (Robson 1993, pp.220–224).

Thus it concerns itself with how safe it is to conclude that the measure undertaken has accounted for the error that is inherent in any observation. Polit and Hungler (1993, pp.244–248) describe three facets for the testing of reliability – stability, internal consistency and equivalence:

- **Stability** is concerned with how well the instrument obtains similar results following repeated measures. It is the external reliability of the measure, or consistency over time (Bryman and Cramer 1997, p.63). The method used for examining this is test–retest reliability, described by Polit and Hungler (1993, p.447) as *'the assessment of the stability of an instrument by correlating the scores obtained on repeated administrations'*. Although this is the chosen method for examining the stability, it does not come without well-acknowledged disadvantages. First, the concept that the instrument is measuring may well differ independently of the stability of the instrument in the intervening period of measures being taken. Second, memory may influence the second measure and despite actual change the correlation coefficient obtained is high. Third, a cursory approach may be used to complete the second measure (or in fact the first): the subject or observer objects to filling a second (or first rating) and thus haphazardly fills in the instrument, resulting in a low correlation coefficient (Robson 1993, pp.220–225).

- **Equivalence** is concerned with the extent to which the instrument can determine consistently the same result for the same subject. The usual method for determining this is inter-rater reliability. Two or more raters assess the same subject at the same time. This is a measure of how closely raters agree in their scoring within a scale.

- **Internal consistency** is when a scale is assumed to measure a single underlying continuum, and its items should be strongly positively related both to each other and to the continuum (Oppenheim 1992, p.160). In order to check this, its homogeneity can be measured using an internal consistency method. The usual method for this is the split-half approach, where half the items on the measure are correlated with the other half to obtain a correlation coefficient. However, the method that has now become the more preferable is Cronbach's Alpha, where all possible alternatives of dividing the scale for the split-half method are correlated. This method gives an indication of the sampling of the items that contribute to the scale.

To be **valid** is to be sound or defensible, and well-grounded (Oxford University Press 1995). In research terms the validity of a measure is concerned with how well it measures the concept that it is supposed to be measuring. Conceptual clarity is a necessary precursor to measurement validity, which can be achieved through rigorous definitions which enable theoretical understanding and consistency of measurement (Moody 1990, pp.250–251).

The relationship between reliability and validity is reciprocal; one cannot exist without the other. However, simply because a measure is reliable it does not follow that it is valid. A measure can be extremely reliable at 'measuring', but not at measuring the concept intended.

A number of established approaches to the examination of validity are available:

- **Face validity** is the extent to which, *prima facie*, the content of the instrument appears to measure the concept under examination.
- **Predictive validity** is the strength of the relationship between the concept being measured and an outcome. Can measure x predict behaviour y?
- **Construct validity** is the extent to which the instrument measures a theoretical construct (e.g. 'risk'). The literature plays a major role in determining this; it is difficult to establish and is related to face, predictive and criterion validity (Robson 1993, p.68).
- **Internal validity** is the extent to which items in the measure offer a synchronous and logical description of the concept under study.
- **Criterion-related validity** is the efficiency with which the instrument operationalises and measures related theoretical constructs.
- **Content validity** is the detailed opinion from experts in the field that the instrument effectively measures the concepts involved.
- **External validity** is the extent to which a positive correlation exists between the measure and other known measures related to its central concepts.

Predictive validity and internal consistency

Item analysis is a test of the predictive validity and internal consistency of an instrument, carried out by measuring the extent to which each item contributes to the scale as a whole (Oppenheim 1992, pp.198–199). It employs a corrected version of an appropriate correlational technique and the score achieved for each individual item is correlated with the total score for the scale, minus the score for that item. The logic is that ideally the score for each item should correlate significantly with the total score for the scale. Thus the correlation achieved by each item is a direct measure of its predictive validity as an appropriate contributor to the scale as a whole.

It should be noted that if, in the early stages of a study, an item or items do not correlate significantly with total scores, this does not necessarily mean that such items are invalid. There are in fact a number of other reasons why this can occur:

- There may be **insufficient data** to reveal a correlation, which may only become evident when more underlying data have been acquired.
- Assessors may be **inexperienced in the use of an instrument**; and particularly in the assessment of those items that do not appear to correlate significantly with the total score.
- For various reasons, assessors **may lack the information necessary** to carry out an effective assessment of such items. This will lead to

increased variability and a loss of obvious pattern in the resultant scores.

- Assessors may lack precise, clear-cut operational definitions for such items; or they may misunderstand such definitions; or they may fail to consult the definitions appropriately whilst carrying out the assessment.

So what can the mental health nurse take from all this? Simply that although instruments should be developed from rigorous research and development focusing heavily on reliability and validity this is not an easy but rather an onerous task for any instrument developer. Hence why some ignore this task at their peril!

Inappropriate use of instruments

Problems associated with inappropriate use of instruments are often worse than not using them at all, both in terms of incorrect interpretation and infringement of copyright or other publisher requirements. Inappropriate use of instruments has further implications which can be serious given that risk management decisions can be taken on the results of such instruments, and litigation becomes a possibility if their application has been erroneous in any way. There is probably the misuse and abuse of screening and assessment instruments taking place on a daily basis in mental health practice. Some of this may be unwittingly and at other times knowingly done. As we will see through the discussion below, this can have serious consequences.

Ignoring copyright

Screening and assessment instruments are subject to copyright for a number of reasons. Foremost has to be so that ownership can be registered and clearly established. Following on from this, the copyright holder may allow someone to freely copy or use the instrument but more usually will expect permission for use to be requested for a number of reasons. This permission may be required because the owner wants to charge to use the instrument and/or wants users to have specific qualifications or training to use it. Some instruments are not formally registered for copyright but are published as part of a journal article, in a book chapter or on the internet. In these cases the journal or book publisher will have to be approached to obtain permission to reproduce the instrument. In the latter case, where an instrument is published on the internet, the same principles apply about asking for permission to use from the author. Therefore, it is important that mental health nurses check out any copyright issues for the instruments they use prior to integrating them into their practice. Failure to follow correct copyright procedures could mean they are open to legal consequences.

'Stealing' the instrument

Using an instrument and passing it off as your own, or integrating this within another instrument without permission from the copyright holder or author, or without reference to the original author, is paramount to 'theft' or plagiarism. The clear message here is that if you want to include an instrument in local assessment documentation you need to get permission to do this. Do not alter the format, unless permission is given, and always cite that permission was given, by whom and when. If an instrument is not restricted via copyright, or you cannot make contact with the copyright holder or author, then you may be able to use it in your documentation if it is not altered *but* check with the Copyright Licensing Agency (http://www.cla.co.uk/) and your legal department at work first.

Altering the scores on instruments

Chapter 3 discussed some of the issues of altering the scores of instruments and the consequences this may have. The reader is directed back to this chapter to clarify these issues.

Adapting the content of instruments

Another important issue is when someone decides to adapt an instrument for use by changing words or concepts contained within the instrument, thus affecting its overall reliability and validity. Furthermore there have been cases where assessment instruments have been adapted, then adapted again and published as another instrument, consequently involving lengthy legal battles as to their real authorship. As we saw above, instruments develop via rigorous means and items contained within them undergo careful scrutiny in relation to their inclusion. Whilst work does go on, and sometimes items do get removed from time to time in revised versions, this is usually following statistical analysis of the items and the relationship to the outcome (risk) measures. Therefore, it is important that mental health nurses do not remove or add items because they think they should be there without first consulting the author(s) of the instrument.

Appropriate training or qualifications

Many instruments require the user to have specific training, qualifications or background information in order to use them. Sometimes they have related manuals to help with the scoring and interpretation of the results. Thus it is important for mental health nurses to be aware of the requirements and not to use instruments without the proper skills, knowledge and training. Again, failure to do this can severely affect the reliability and validity of the results.

Using instruments for purposes other than what they were designed for

As has been discussed in the previous section, instrument development entails significant work and validation, often involving years of work. Many assessment instruments are designed for use with specific populations and if used in other populations their reliability and validity can be questionable.

Hoffmann and Shulman (2005) writing on a website discuss eloquently how easily instrument abuse can occur and good tools used badly can harm clients. Typically they highlight through examples from freely available substance abuse assessment how this takes the form of using the instrument for purposes or with populations for which it is not designed. Quoting these two authors:

'In some cases, this results from the confusion between assessment functions such as screening vs. determining a diagnosis. In other cases, the problem may stem from a failure to understand the appropriate uses for which a given instrument is designed, such as using a program evaluation tool for conducting a clinical intake. This problem takes on its most egregious forms when a particular instrument is mandated for an inappropriate use. One of the classic and pervasive misuses of instruments consists of using screens instead of diagnostic instruments for clinical intakes and treatment planning. This would be analogous to an oncologist using results from a mammogram or colonoscopy in recommending a mastectomy or colon surgery for a possible malignancy, instead of using a definitive biopsy for developing the treatment plan. The proper function of a screen is to determine level of risk for a given condition. A screen is basically a quick, easily administered and inexpensive means of identifying the probability that an individual is likely to have a given condition or disorder. This is sometimes referred to as "ruling in" (likely that the individual has the specified condition or disorder) or "ruling out" (unlikely that the individual has the specified condition or disorder). If the condition is "ruled in," further assessment is required to make a definitive determination of whether or not an individual actually has the condition in question.'

In their conclusion to this short article they sum up issues in a clear message that mental health nurses need to bear in mind:

'By now, it should be abundantly clear that "instrument abuse" can occur through the inappropriate use of good tools. Misuse of assessment instruments can have serious consequences for those afflicted with substance use disorders and those professionals providing treatment services. Instrument abuse can result in inappropriate care for the client and may expose the clinician to professional liability claims' (Hoffmann and Shulman 2005).

So to conclude this section, the key message for mental health nurses in relation to instrument use is to be careful they have permission to use an unaltered instrument that they have the skills, knowledge and ability to use. Failure to do so can affect the reliability and validity of their findings, result in reduced patient outcome and could make them open to criticism or liability.

Some specific risk assessment instruments that mental health nurses could utilise

It is clear from this chapter and others in this book that there are many instruments that mental health nurses can utilise to support their risk assessments. The sample of instruments that follow are merely intended to highlight some of those that are available for mental health nurses to use to support their clinical practice. None is specifically suggested and it is up to individual practitioners to decide if and how they meet their needs and of course if they have the relevant training and experience to utilise them effectively.

General and multiple risk

There are many instruments that could be considered to assist in the assessment of general risk in those individuals with mental health problems. Not to go into any real depth, these include:

- the Brief Psychiatric Rating Scale (BPRS) (Overall and Gorham 1962);
- the Symptom Checklist-90-Revised (SCL-90–R) (Derogatis 1992); and
- the whole other array of scales that are available to measure delusions, hallucinations, fear, anxiety, etc.

It also includes those that focus on more specific multiple risks. For example:

- the Short-Term Assessment of Risk and Treatability (START) (Webster *et al.* 2004);
- the Behavioural Status Index (BEST-Index) (Reed and Woods 2000).

The START (Webster *et al.* 2004) contains 20 items that are considered around seven risk domains:

1. violence to others;
2. suicide;
3. self-harm;
4. self-neglect;
5. unauthorised absence;
6. substance use;
7. victimisation.

It also allows the rater to record case-specific risk factors. Both patient strengths and vulnerabilities are recorded on a three-point scale (not present, possibly present, present), and key or critical items highlighted in relation to the 20 given and case-specific items. For one of the items (relationships) a yes or no evaluation of therapeutic alliance is made. For another item (social support) positive peer support is also evaluated as yes or no. Specific risk estimates around the seven risk domains are made (low, moderate or high), as well as T.H.R.E.A.T. (Threats of Harm that are Real, Enactable, Acute and Targetable (Webster *et al.* 2004, p.34)) assessment of violence to others, suicide and self-harm. For each of these seven domains there is also a place to highlight if historical data are available. Current management measures, health concerns and risk formulation are also recorded.

The START is intended for use by all disciplines and items are assessed according to succinct descriptions provided in the published manual. The START can be used with adults with mental, personality and substance-related disorders, in inpatient and community psychiatric, forensic, and correctional populations. Research surrounding the START is still developing, but initial studies indicate good psychometric properties. There is extensive interest in the instrument. Box 4.1 contains the details of the START items, training requirements, availability and access details and some related references.

The Behavioural Status Index (BEST-Index) (Reed and Woods 2000) evaluates life skills, social risk and related daily behaviours. The BEST-Index consists of six subscales:

1. social risk;
2. insight;
3. communication and social skills;
4. work and recreational activities;
5. self and family care;
6. empathy.

Box 4.1   Short-Term Assessment of Risk and Treatability (START) (Webster *et al.* 2004).

Items:

- Social skills
- Relationships
- Occupational
- Recreational
- Self-care
- Mental state
- Emotional state
- Substance use
- Impulse control
- External triggers

- Social support
- Material resources
- Attitudes
- Medication adherence
- Rule adherence
- Conduct
- Insight
- Plans
- Coping
- Treatability

Training requirements
A structured education and training programme is encouraged by the authors for all staff involved in using the START. A trainer's manual is available (see Desmarais *et al.* 2006 in related references).

Availability and access
The START is available for purchase from http://www.bcmhas.ca/Research/Research_START.htm. Email: start@forensic.bc.ca.

Related references
Desmarais, S.L., Webster, C.D., Martin, M.L., Dassinger, C., Brink, J. & Nicholls, T.L. (2006) *Manual for the Short-Term Assessment of Risk and Treatability (START): Instructors' Guide and Workbook* (Version 2). St. Joseph's Healthcare, Hamilton, Ontario, and Forensic Psychiatric Services Commission, Port Coquitlam, British Columbia.

Nicholls, T.L., Brink, J., Desmarais, S.L., Webster, C.D. & Martin, M.L. (2006). The Short-Term Assessment of Risk and Treatability (START): a prospective validation study in a forensic psychiatric sample. *Assessment*, **13**(3), 313–327.

Webster, C.D., Nicholls, T.L., Martin, M.L., Desmarais, S.L. & Brink, J. (2006). Short-Term Assessment of Risk and Treatability (START): the case for a new structured professional judgement scheme. *Behavioral Sciences and the Law*, **24**, 747–766.

These identify essential components of human social behaviour:

- The social risk sub-scale contains 20 items measuring constructs commonly associated with risk: for example, overt and covert violence to the more generally disruptive behaviours.
- The insight sub-scale again consists of 20 items and examines an individual's cognitive constructs of reality.

- The communication and social skills sub-scale consists of 30 items. Principally examined are behaviours of the social skills type or adaptive social behaviours.
- The work and recreational activities sub-scale consists of 20 items. Here, paid work is not necessarily a feature and the section is concerned with those constructive activities with which a wide range of individuals could identify.
- The self and family care sub-scale consists of 30 items and measures such daily and socially important areas as personal hygiene, cooking skills and other aspects of self-care, care for other members of the family or group, and family-group relationships.
- The empathy sub-scale consists of 30 items and is designed to assess the capacity of patients to empathise with others, more especially with those who have been victimised.

All 150 items that make up the BEST-Index are scored using a stepwise approach from 1 (worst case) through 5 (best case). The logic here is that functioning is viewed within a normative, rather than a sociopathic, frame of reference: consequently a higher score indicates the achievement of a more socially adaptive or behavioural performance that would be viewed as 'socially acceptable' by others in the contexts of the patient's family, social and cultural networks. As lower scores are indicative of poor functioning or problematic areas, these should be the main focus of concern. There is extensive interest in the instrument. Box 4.2 contains details of the BEST-Index items, training requirements, availability and access details and some related references.

Risk to others

Probably not surprising there have been many instruments developed to help in the assessment of risk to others, with the most prolific work done around sexual offending and violence risk. A few examples in relation to violence to others are:

- the Historical Clinical Risk-20 (HCR-20) (Webster *et al.* 1997);
- the Violence Risk Appraisal Guide (VRAG) (Quinsey *et al.* 1998);
- the Violence Risk Scale (VRS) (Wong and Gordon 2000);
- the Brøset Violence Checklist (BVC) (Almvik and Woods 1998).

For sexual offence risk some examples are:

- the Sex Offender Risk Appraisal Guide (SORAG) (Quinsey *et al.* 1998);
- the Rapid Risk Assessment for Sexual Violence (RRASOR) (Hanson 1997);

Box 4.2   Behavioural Status Index (BEST-Index) (Reed and Woods 2000).

Risk sub-scale items

- Family support
- Serious violence to others without apparent trigger event
- Serious violence to others following trigger event
- Minor violence to others without apparent trigger event
- Minor violence to others following trigger event
- Serious self harm
- Superficial self harm
- Verbal aggression without apparent trigger event
- Verbal aggression following trigger event
- Attacks on objects without apparent trigger event
- Attacks on objects following trigger event
- Breaches of security
- Disruptive episodes
- Imitative disruption
- Inappropriate sexual behaviours
- Sado-masochistic behaviours
- Macho gear and adornment
- Obsessive-compulsive behaviours
- Substance abuse
- Psychiatric disturbance

Insight sub-scale items

- Awareness of tension
- Description of tension
- Tension-reducing strategies
- Recognition of negative or angry feelings
- Tension-producing thoughts
- Tension-producing events
- Personal strategy for reducing tension
- Identifying relaxing thoughts
- Identifying relaxing activities
- Attributes disliked in others
- Attributes liked in others
- Events producing insecurity
- Events producing security
- Antecedent events leading to treatment
- Ascription of responsibility
- Self-appraisal
- Prioritisation of problems
- Goal-planning
- Compliance with therapy
- Expectations

Communication and social skills sub-scale items

- Facial expression
- Eye contact
- Orientation to others
- Body posture
- Expressive gestures
- Social distance
- Tone of voice
- Voice modulation
- Verbal delivery
- Conversational initiative
- Amount of speech
- Fluency

Work and recreational activities sub-scale items

- Attendance
- Timekeeping
- Sickness absence
- Adaptability
- Concentration
- Team work
- Interest
- Quality of work
- Initiative
- Responsiveness
- Leisure pursuits
- Leisure and relaxation

- Turn-taking
- Listening skills
- Response to questions
- Conversational topics
- Egocentric conversation
- Frankness
- Expressing opinions
- Disagreement
- Arguments
- Making requests
- Assertiveness
- Self-presentation
- Social activities
- Emotional control
- Relationship with others
- Ease of communication
- Sociability and support
- Deferring to others

- Planning leisure activities
- Suitability of selection
- Participation in leisure
- Hobbies and interests
- Interest in shared leisure
- Motivation to shared leisure
- Gender interaction
- Potential sexual partners

Self and family care sub-scale items

- Nutrition
- Cooking
- Eating regularly
- Preparing own meals
- Preparing meals for others
- Storing food
- Stock of food
- Personal hygiene
- Health precautions
- Seeking medical help
- Dressing for weather
- Clothing and footwear
- Caring for clothes
- Storing clothes
- Household dangers
- Managing money
- Economy with resources
- Caring for the home
- Clearing-up after meals
- Washing up
- Making bed(s)
- Changing bed linen
- Going out
- Using public or personal transport
- Shopping
- Personal grooming
- Facial care

Empathy sub-scale items

- Imagining oneself in the life-world of another person
- Understanding the feelings of another person, distinct from those of oneself
- Sensitivity to others
- Expressing sympathy for the wishes and needs of another person
- Pleased for others
- Allows others to express themselves
- Interest in social 'give-and-take'
- Dealing with conflict
- Sharing conversations
- Curbing self-interest
- Listening to others
- Physical 'mirror responses'
- Offering support
- Avoiding abuse
- Listening and questioning
- Making excuses
- Accepting ideas
- Comforting others
- Acknowledging the victim
- Giving others 'breathing space'
- The victim as a person
- Concern for others' troubles
- Psychological 'intrusion'

Box 4.2 Behavioural Status Index (BEST-Index) (Reed and Woods 2000). (*continued*)

● Dressing for the occasion	● Sharing 'terrors'
● Eating out	● Expressing consideration
● Behaviour at table	● Taking an interest
	● Asking about feelings
	● Making eye contact
	● Balancing interests
	● Doing things for others

Training requirements
A training programme has been developed by the authors for those wishing to use it.

Availability and access
The BEST-Index is available from the authors. Email: Dr Val Reed (vreed52@aol.com) or Dr Phil Woods (phil.woods@usask.ca).

Related references
Ross, T., Woods, P., Reed, V., *et al.* (2007) Selecting and monitoring living skills in forensic mental health care: cross-border validation of the BEST-Index. *International Journal of Mental Health*, **36**(4), 3–17.

Woods, P., Reed, V. & Robinson, D. (1999) The Behavioral Status Index: therapeutic assessment of risk, insight and social skills. *Journal of Psychiatric and Mental Health Nursing*, **6**(2), 79–90.

Woods, P., Reed, V. & Collins, M. (2005) The Behavioural Status Index: testing a social risk assessment model in a high security forensic setting. *Journal of Forensic Nursing*, **1**(1), 9–19.

- the Static-99 (Hanson and Thornton 1999);
- the Sexual Violence Risk-20 (SVR-20) (Boer *et al.* 1998);
- the Risk Matrix 2000 (RM 2000) (Hanson and Thornton 2000);
- the Sex Offender Need Assessment Rating (SONAR) (Hanson and Harris 2000);
- the Violence Risk Scale: Sexual Offenders (VRS:SO) (Wong *et al.* 2003).

Some instruments have developed around spousal assault. For example:

- the Spousal Assault Risk Assessment Guide (SARA) (Kropp *et al.* 1999);
- the Brief Spousal Assault Form for the Evaluation of Risk (B-SAFER) (Kropp and Hart 2004).

Others have developed around the assessment of anger and the best known is probably the State-Trait Anger Expression Inventory-2 (STAXI-2)

(Spielberger 1999). One instrument that was not specifically developed for violence risk assessment has served well in the prediction of this: the Psychopathy Checklist-Revised (PCL-R) (Hare 1991, 2003).

Finally some instruments have developed around the measurement of aggression once incidents have occurred. For instance:

- the Overt Aggression Scale (OAS) (Yudofsky *et al.* 1986);
- the Modified Overt Aggression Scale (MOAS) (Kay *et al.* 1988);
- the Staff Observation Aggression Scale-Revised (SOAS-R) (Nijman *et al.* 1999a, b);
- the Report Form for Aggressive Episodes (REFA) (Bjørkly 1996);
- the Rating Scale for Aggression in the Elderly (RAGE) (Patel and Hope 1992);
- the Brief Agitation Rating Scale (BARS) (Finkel *et al.* 1993);
- the Cohen-Mansfield Agitation Inventory (CMAI) (Cohen-Mansfield 1986);
- the Attempted and Actual Assault Scale (ATTACKS) (Bowers *et al.* 2007).

Three of the instruments that have received most attention in the nursing literature will be discussed in more detail.

The HCR-20 (Webster *et al.* 1997) is probably one of the most widely used assessments of future violent behaviour in clinical practice and was developed from an extensive literature review and input from clinicians experienced in forensic psychiatry. It has been the focus of extensive research to date and its psychometric properties are good. The HCR-20 contains 20 items which are divided into three key areas:

- historical (10 items);
- clinical (5 items);
- risk management (5 items).

HCR-20 items are recorded on a three-point scale (absent, possibly present, definitely present), and key or critical items highlighted in relation to the 20 given and case-specific items. The historical items are intended to be an anchor for the risk assessment, with repeated measures taken on the clinical and risk items over periods of time. There is also a final level of risk judgment that is made (low, moderate or high) and this should be based on a careful consideration of the ratings given for the 20 items. The HCR-20 is intended for use by all disciplines to assess both criminal and psychiatric populations. The items are assessed according to in-depth descriptions provided in the published manual. Box 4.3 contains details of the HCR-20 items, training requirements, availability and access details and some related references.

The BVC (Almvik and Woods 1998) is a short-term violence prediction instrument that developed from previous empirical work. Each of the six behaviours are scored for their presence (1) or absence (0). For well-known patients an increase in the behaviour described in Box 4.3 is scored as 1, whereas the habitual behaviour while being non-violent is scored as 0. Clear definitions of behaviours are provided by the authors. Scoring is done by summing the scores for each of the six behaviours. Interpretation of the summed scores is given by the authors as:

0	the risk of violence is small;
1–2	the risk of violence is moderate (preventive measures should be taken);
2 or above	the risk of violence is very high (preventive measures should be taken and plans should be developed to manage the potential violence).

From research studies that are available the BVC appears to have satisfactory psychometric properties and discriminates the violent from not violent

Box 4.3   Historical Clinical Risk-20 (HCR-20) (Webster *et al.* 1997).

Items

Historical

- Previous violence
- Young age at first violent incident
- Relationship instability
- Employment problems
- Substance use problems
- Major mental illness
- Psychopathy
- Early maladjustment
- Personality disorder
- Prior supervision failure

Clinical

- Lack of insight
- Negative attitudes
- Active symptoms of major mental illness
- Impulsivity
- Unresponsive to treatment

Risk

- Plans lack feasibility
- Exposure to destabilisers
- Lack of personal support
- Non-compliance with remediation attempts
- Stress

Training

The HCR-20 website states a degree, certificate or licence to practice in a healthcare profession (this includes nursing) plus appropriate training and experience in the ethical administration, scoring and interpretation of clinical behavioural assessment instruments. Certified trainers are available in many countries. It should also be borne in mind that full completion of the assessment requires a PCL-R rating to be taken which needs specific in-depth education. Nurses that do use the HCR-20 often omit the rating for psychopathy.

Availability and access

The HCR-20 is available for purchase from http://www3.parinc.com/products/product.aspx?Productid=HCR-20.

Related references

(Note this is merely a sample of some of those available that the chapter authors have found useful. A literature search will result in many more)

Belfrage, H. (1998) Implementing the HCR-20 scheme for risk assessment in a forensic psychiatric hospital: integrating research and clinical practice. *Journal of Forensic Psychiatry*, **9**, 328–338.

Belfrage, H., Fransson, R. & Strand, S. (2000) Prediction of violence using the HCR-20: a prospective study in two maximum-security correctional institutions. *Journal of Forensic Psychiatry*, **11**, 167–175.

Dolan, M. & Doyle, M. (2000) Violence risk prediction. *British Journal of Psychiatry*, **177**, 303–311.

Dolan, M. & Khawaja, A. (2004) The HCR-20 and post-discharge outcome in male patients discharged from medium security in the UK. *Aggressive Behaviour*, **30**, 469–483.

Watt, W., Topping-Morris, B., Doyle, M. & Mason, T. (2003) Pre-admission nursing assessments in a Welsh medium secure unit (1991–2000). Part 2. Comparison of traditional nursing assessment with the HCR-20 risk assessment tool. *International Journal of Nursing Studies*, **40**, 657–662.

over the next 24-hour period. Box 4.4 contains details of the BVC items, training requirements, availability and access details and some related references.

The SOAS-R (Nijman *et al.* 1999a, b) is widely used in research and clinical practice as an incident reporting and analysis measure. The SOAS-R through many studies has been reported to have adequate psychometric properties and to be clinically useful. Box 4.5 details the SOAS-R items, training requirements, availability and access details and some related references.

Risk to self

Many scales have been developed to help screen and assess for suicide, self-harm and self-neglect. For example, in relation to suicide:

- the Beck Hopelessness Scale (BHS) (Beck *et al.* 1974a);
- the Scale for Suicide Ideation (SSI) (Beck and Steer 1991);
- the Suicide Intent Scales (SIS) (Beck *et al.* 1974b);
- the revised SIS (Pierce 1977, 1981);
- SAD PERSONS (Patterson *et al.* 1983);

Box 4.4   Brøset Violence Checklist (BVC) (Almvik and Woods 1998).

The BVC behaviours are:

- Confusion
- Irritability
- Boisterousness
- Physical threats
- Verbal threats
- Attacks on objects.

Training
No specific training is necessary, but some training materials are available from the authors if required.

Availability and access
The BVC is available from the authors. Email: Dr Roger Almvik (roger.almvik@ntnu.no) or Dr Phil Woods (phil.woods@usask.ca). Although the BVC is copyrighted, permission is always provided for use providing the original source is cited. An electronic version is also available for purchase from http://www.igcn.nl/?p=63&PHPSESSID=3ca87ea52b2e8efe161bcff230a1856f.

Related references
Abderhalden, C., Needham, I., Miserez, B., Almvik, R., Dassen, T., Haug, H.J. & Fischer, J.E. (2004) Predicting inpatient violence in acute psychiatric wards using the Brøset-Violence-Checklist: a multicentre prospective cohort study. *Journal of Psychiatric and Mental Health Nursing*, **11**(4), 422–427.

Almvik, R., Woods, P. & Rasmussen, K. (2000) The Brøset Violence Checklist (BVC): sensitivity, specificity and inter-rater reliability. *Journal of Interpersonal Violence*, **15**(12), 1284–1296.

Almvik, R., Woods, P. & Rasmussen, K. (2007) Assessing risk for imminent violence in the elderly: the Brøset Violence Checklist. *International Journal of Geriatric Psychiatry*, **22**(9), 862–867.

Björkdahl, A., Olsson, D. & Palmstierna, T. (2006) Nurses' short-term prediction of violence in acute psychiatric intensive care. *Acta Psychiatrica Scandinavica*, **113**(3), 224–229.

Woods, P., Ashley, C., Kayto, D. & Heusdens, C. (2008) Piloting violence and incident reporting measures on one acute mental health inpatient unit. *Issues in Mental Health Nursing*, **29**(5), 455–469.

Box 4.5 Staff Observation and Aggression Scale-Revised (SOAS-R) (Nijman *et al.* 1999a, b).

The SOAS-R developed from the original SOAS following extensive empirical work. This revision involved some adjustments to the format and more fine-grained severity scoring system. The SOAS-R consists of five columns, each pertaining to specific aspects of the incident. According to the authors the first and last columns describe the immediate cause and the measures used to stop the aggression (i.e. provocation and measure(s) to stop aggression) and the other three columns describe the central aspects of the aggression (i.e. means used by the patient, target of aggression; consequence(s) for victim).

The severity scores for the SOAS-R can range from 0 to 22 points, with higher scores indicating more severity. Nijman *et al.* (1999) suggest a classification into mild (scores ranging from 0 to 7), moderate (scores ranging from 8 to 15) and severe (scores ranging from 16 to 22). However, Nijman *et al.* (1999) did caution on using this new scoring system outside of aggression that is outwardly directed, as their study of aggression directed towards self using the SOAS-R was based on a small sample size.

Training
No specific training is required.

Availability and access
The SOAS-R is available in Nijman *et al.* (1999a, b). Please contact the authors for permission to use. An electronic version is also available for purchase from http://www.soas-r.com/uk/home.html and http://www.igcn.nl/?p=39&PHPSESSID= 3ca87ea52b2e8efe161bcff230a1856f.

Related references
Nijman, H., Evers, C., Merckelbach, H. & Palmstierna, T. (2002) Assessing aggression severity with the revised staff observation aggression scale. *Journal of Nervous and Mental Disease*, **190**(3), 198–200.

Nijman, H.L., Palmstierna, T., Almvik, R. & Stolker, J.J. (2005) Fifteen years of research with the Staff Observation Aggression Scale: a review. *Acta Psychiatrica Scandinavica*, **111**(1), 12–21.

Palmstierna, T. & Wistedt, B. (1987) Staff observation aggression scale, SOAS: presentation and evaluation. *Acta Psychiatrica Scandinavica*, **76**(6), 657–663.

- the Nurses' Global Assessment of Suicide Risk (NGASR) (Cutliffe and Barker 2004).

Some self-injury scales can be found but not in abundance, for example:

- the self-report Self-Injury Motivation Scale (SIMS) (Osuch *et al.* 1999; Osuch, undated);
- the self report Self-Injury Questionnaire (SIQ) (Alexander 1999; see also Santa Mina *et al.* 2006).

Sub-scales from such instruments as the Behavioural Status Index (BEST-Index) (Reed and Woods 2000) can help to assess risk of self-neglect.

The Beck Hopelessness Scale (BHS) (Beck *et al.* 1974a) is a self-report screening measure of negative attitudes about the future during the past week. It can also be verbally administered by someone who is trained for the purpose. The original intention behind the BHS was to predict who would or would not commit suicide in adults. The BHS contains 20 true/false items around three major aspects of hopelessness:

- feelings about the future;
- loss of motivation;
- expectations.

Scoring is very straightforward and each of the items are scored as 0 or 1. A total score is then calculated by summing all the pessimistic responses. Although the manual contains general cut-off guidelines, these need to be considered in the context of clinical presentation as well (Beck and Steer 1988). The BHS has been found in many studies to have adequate psychometric properties. The BHS can be obtained from the publisher at http://www.pearson-uk.com/product.aspx?n=1316&s=1322&cat=1426&skey=2647.

The Scale for Suicide Ideation (SSI) (Beck and Steer 1991) is a self-report measure for detecting and measuring the current intensity of specific attitudes, behaviours and plans to commit suicide during the past week. It can also be verbally administered by someone who is trained for the purpose. It is the same measure that is referred to as the Beck Scale for Suicide Ideation. The SSI contains 21 items. The first 19 items have three options (0–2) and are scored in relation to the intensity of the suicidality: for instance:

- wish to die;
- desire to make an active or passive suicide attempt;
- duration and frequency of ideation;
- sense of control over making an attempt;
- number of deterrents;
- amount of actual preparation for a contemplated attempt.

The score is then summed. The remaining two items assess the number of previous suicide attempts and the seriousness of the intent to die associated with the last attempt. The first five items can be viewed as a screening measure. The SSI has been found in many studies to have adequate psychometric properties. The SSI can be obtained from the publisher at http://www.pearson-uk.com/product.aspx?n=1316&s=1322&cat=1426&skey=2649.

The Suicide Intent Scales (SIS) (Beck *et al.* 1974b) were developed to assess patients who attempt suicide but survive, and are widely used in clinical practice around the world. Pierce (1977, 1981) developed and validated a modified version of the SIS. The original SIS (Beck *et al.* 1974b) contains 20 items scored on a three-point scale (1–3). Box 4.6 contains details of the SIS items, training requirements, and availability and access details. The revised SIS (Pierce 1977, 1981) contains 12 items scored on a three-point scale (0–2), except premeditation which is scored on a four-point scale (0–3). Box 4.7 contains details of the revised SIS items, training requirements, and availability and access details.

Risk of substance abuse

As discussed later in Chapter 7, risk of substance abuse will involve a more detailed assessment of risk, often using lengthy interviews. However, many screening instruments have been developed to assist in identifying those most at risk of either developing abuse or already abusing. In this chapter, four of these are identified:

- the CAGE (Ewing 1984);
- the Drug Abuse Screening Test (DAST) (Gavin *et al.* 1989);
- the Michigan Alcohol Screening Test (MAST) (Selzer 1971);
- the Alcohol Use Disorders Identification Test (AUDIT) (developed by the World Health Organisation; the currently available manual is Babor *et al.* (2001)).

These are user friendly and readily available for use on the internet, as either self-administered or clinically administered instruments.

Box 4.8 reports details of the CAGE items, training requirements, and availability and access details.

Box 4.9 reports details of the DAST items, training requirements, and availability and access details.

Box 4.10 reports details of the MAST items, training requirements, availability and access details and some related references.

Box 4.11 reports details of the AUDIT items, training requirements, and availability and access.

Box 4.6   Suicide Intent Scale (SIS) (Beck *et al.* 1974b).

The SIS contains the following 20 items scored on a scale of 1–3:

Objective circumstances related to suicide attempt

- Isolation
- Timing
- Precautions against discovery/intervention
- Acting to get help during/after attempt
- Final acts in anticipation of death (will, gifts, insurance)
- Active preparation for attempt
- Suicide note
- Overt communication of intent before the attempt

Self report

- Alleged purpose of attempt
- Expectations of fatality
- Conception of method's lethality
- Seriousness of attempt
- Attitude toward living/dying
- Conception of medical rescuability
- Degree of premeditation

Other aspects (not included in total score)

- Reaction to attempt
- Visualisation of death
- Number of previous attempts
- Relationship between alcohol intake and attempt
- Relationship between drug intake and attempt

Source: http://everything2.com/index.pl?node_id=1318146.

Only the first 15 items are summed and count towards the overall risk score. Scores can range from 15 to 45. Total scores of 15–19 indicate low intent; scores of 20–28 medium intent; and scores of 29 or greater high intent. From research studies that are available the SIS appears to have satisfactory psychometric properties.

Training
No training details are available on the SIS.

Availability and access
The SIS is readily available on many websites. As far as the chapter authors are aware it is not copyrighted, providing the original source is cited.

Box 4.7   The revised SIS (Pierce 1977, 1981).

The revised SIS contains the following 15 items scored on a scale of 0–2, except premeditation which is scored on a scale of 0–3:

Circumstances score

- Isolation
- Timing
- Precautions against rescue
- Acting to gain help
- Final acts in anticipation
- Suicide note

Self report score

- Lethality
- Stated intent
- Premeditation
- Reaction to act

Medical risk score

- Predictable outcome
- Death without medical treatment

Source: http://www.patient.co.uk/showdoc/40024821/.

All 12 items are summed and count towards the overall risk score. Scores can range from 0 to 25. Total scores of less than 3 indicate low risk; scores of 4–10 medium risk; and scores of 11 or greater high risk. From research studies that are available the revised SIS appears to have satisfactory psychometric properties.

Training
No training details are available on the revised SIS.

Availability and access
The revised SIS is readily available on many websites. As far as the chapter authors are aware it is not copyrighted, providing the original source is cited.

Box 4.8   CAGE (Ewing 1984).

The CAGE is a simple four question (yes or no) screening test to identify use or abuse of alcohol over the user's lifetime. The four questions, from whence the acronym CAGE comes from (see italicised words), are:

1.   Have you ever felt you ought to *cut* down on your drinking?
2.   Have you ever felt *annoyed* by people criticising your drinking?
3.   Have you ever felt bad or *guilty* about drinking?
4.   Have you ever had a drink first thing in the morning (*eye*-opener)?

Scoring is done by allocating 1 point to each 'yes' answer. Total scores of 2 or above are thought to be clinically significant and may indicate alcohol dependence. Further assessment should be undertaken to determine if this is the case. Although the original research was undertaken on a small sample, subsequent clinical research has found the CAGE to be a useful screening tool.

Training
No training is required and the CAGE can be self-administered.

Availability and access
The CAGE is readily available on many websites and within mental health nursing textbooks. As far as the chapter authors are aware it is not copyrighted, providing the original source is cited.

Box 4.9   Drug Abuse Screening Test (DAST) (Gavin *et al.* 1989).

The DAST is a simple 28 question (yes or no) screening test to identify use or abuse of drugs over the last 12 months. This test specifically does not include alcohol use. The 28 questions are:

1.   Have you used drugs other than those required for medical reasons?
2.   Have you abused prescription drugs?
3.   Do you abuse more than one drug at a time?
4.   Can you get through the week without using drugs (other than those required for medical reasons)?
5.   Are you always able to stop using drugs when you want to?
6.   Do you abuse drugs on a continuous basis?
7.   Do you try to limit your drug use to certain situations?
8.   Have you had 'blackouts' or 'flashbacks' as a result of drug use?
9.   Do you ever feel bad about your drug abuse?
10.   Does your spouse (or parents) ever complain about your involvement with drugs?

11. Do your friends or relatives know or suspect you abuse drugs?
12. Has drug abuse ever created problems between you and your spouse?
13. Has any family member ever sought help for problems related to your drug use?
14. Have you ever lost friends because of your use of drugs?
15. Have you ever neglected your family or missed work because of your use of drugs?
16. Have you ever been in trouble at work because of drug abuse?
17. Have you ever lost a job because of drug abuse?
18. Have you gotten into fights when under the influence of drugs?
19. Have you ever been arrested because of unusual behaviour while under the influence of drugs?
20. Have you ever been arrested for driving while under the influence of drugs?
21. Have you engaged in illegal activities to obtain drugs?
22. Have you ever been arrested for possession of illegal drugs?
23. Have you ever experienced withdrawal symptoms as a result of heavy drug intake?
24. Have you had medical problems as a result of your drug use (e.g. memory loss, hepatitis, convulsions or bleeding)?
25. Have you ever gone to anyone for help for a drug problem?
26. Have you ever been in hospital for medical problems related to your drug use?
27. Have you ever been involved in a treatment programme specifically related to drug use?
28. Have you been treated as an outpatient for problems related to drug abuse?

Scoring is done by allocating 1 point to each 'yes' answer, except for questions 4 and 5 where 1 point is allocated for a 'no' answer. Total scores of 6 or above are thought to be clinically significant and may indicate a substance use problem. Further assessment should be undertaken to determine if this is the case. From research studies that are available the DAST appears to have satisfactory psychometric properties.

Training
No training is required and the DAST can be self-administered.

Availability and access
The DAST is readily available on many websites and within mental health nursing textbooks. Some of these websites use a 20-item revised version. As far as the chapter authors are aware it is not copyrighted, providing the original source is cited.

Box 4.10   Michigan Alcohol Screening Test (MAST) (Selzer 1971).

Most versions of the MAST are the simple 22 question (yes or no) self-administered screening test to identify use or abuse of alcohol over the user's lifetime. The original version had 25 questions and used a more complex scoring method. The 22 questions are:

1. Do you feel you are a normal drinker ('normal' is defined as drinking as much or less than most other people)?
2. Have you ever awakened the morning after drinking the night before and found that you could not remember a part of the evening?
3. Does any near relative or close friend ever worry or complain about your drinking?
4. Can you stop drinking without difficulty after one or two drinks?
5. Do you ever feel guilty about your drinking?
6. Have you ever attended a meeting of Alcoholics Anonymous (AA)?
7. Have you ever gotten into physical fights when drinking?
8. Has drinking ever created problems between you and a near relative or close friend?
9. Has any family member or close friend gone to anyone for help about your drinking?
10. Have you ever lost friends because of your drinking?
11. Have you ever gotten into trouble at work because of drinking?
12. Have you ever lost a job because of drinking?
13. Have you ever neglected your obligations, family or work for two or more days in a row because you were drinking?
14. Do you drink before noon fairly often?
15. Have you ever been told you have liver trouble, such as cirrhosis?
16. After heavy drinking, have you ever had delirium tremens (DTs), severe shaking, or visual or auditory (hearing) hallucinations?
17. Have you ever gone to anyone for help about your drinking?
18. Have you ever been hospitalised because of drinking?
19. Has your drinking ever resulted in your being hospitalised in a psychiatric ward?
20. Have you ever gone to any doctor, social worker, clergyman or mental health clinic for help with any emotional problem in which drinking was part of the problem?
21. Have you been arrested more than once for driving under the influence of alcohol?
22. Have you ever been arrested, or detained by an official for a few hours, because of other behaviour while drinking?

Scoring is done by allocating 1 point if the answer was 'no' to questions 1 and 4. Score 1 point if the answer was 'yes' to questions 2, 3 or 5 through 22. A total score of 6 or above indicates hazardous drinking and further assessment should be undertaken to determine if this is the case. From research studies that are available the MAST appears to have satisfactory psychometric properties.

Training
No training is required and the MAST can be self-administered.

Availability and access
The MAST is readily available on many websites and within mental health nursing textbooks. As far as the chapter authors are aware it is not copyrighted, providing the original source is cited.

Related references
Bradley, K.A., Boyd-Wickizer, J., Powell, S.H. & Burman, M.L. (1998) Alcohol screening questionnaires in women: a critical review. *Journal of the American Medical Association*, **280**(2), 166–171.

Hirata, E.S., Almeida, O.P., Funari, R.R. & Klein, E.L. (2001) Validity of the Michigan Alcoholism Screening Test (MAST) for the detection of alcohol-related problems among male geriatric outpatients. *American Journal of Geriatric Psychiatry*, **9**, 30–34.

Maisto, S.A., Connors, G.J. & Allen, J.P. (1995) Contrasting self-report screens for alcohol problems: a review. *Alcoholism: Clinical and Experimental Research*, **19**(6), 1510–1516.

Teitelbaum, L. & Mullen, B. (2000) Validity of the MAST in psychiatric settings: a META-analytic integration. *Journal of Studies on Alcohol*, **61**(2), 254–261.

Box 4.11 Alcohol Use Disorders Identification Test (AUDIT) (developed by the World Health Organisation; Barbor *et al.* 2001).

The AUDIT was developed by WHO in the early 1980s and the current available manual is Babor *et al.* (2001). It contains 10 questions that can be administered either as an interview or as a self-report questionnaire and reflect alcohol use of the previous 12 months. Each question has a range of responses from 0–4. The questions are:

1. How often do you have a drink containing alcohol?
2. How many drinks containing alcohol do you have on a typical day when you are drinking?
3. How often do you have six or more drinks on one occasion?
4. How often during the last year have you found that you were not able to stop drinking once you had started?
5. How often during the last year have you failed to do what was normally expected from you because of drinking?
6. How often during the last year have you been unable to remember what happened the night before because you had been drinking?
7. How often during the last year have you needed an alcoholic drink first thing in the morning to get yourself going after a night of heavy drinking?

Box 4.11   Alcohol Use Disorders Identification Test (AUDIT) (developed by the World Health Organisation; Barbor *et al.* 2001). (*continued*)

---

8. How often during the last year have you had a feeling of guilt or remorse after drinking?
9. Have you or someone else been injured as a result of your drinking?
10. Has a relative, friend, doctor or another health professional expressed concern about your drinking or suggested you cut down?

Scoring is done by totaling the relative score from 0–4 for each answer given to these questions. Total scores of 8 or above in men (7 in women and men over 65) indicate hazardous drinking and further assessment should be undertaken to determine if this is the case. The manual suggests further interpretation of scores based on research studies undertaken. From research studies that are available the AUDIT appears to have satisfactory psychometric properties.

Training
No training is required and the AUDIT can be self-administered.

Availability and access
The AUDIT is readily available on many websites. The manual also has versions for clinical use. As far as the chapter authors are aware it is not copyrighted, providing the original source is cited.

Conclusion

As discussed in Chapters 2 and 3, risk assessment and management in mental health practice is moving in the direction of structured clinical judgment. This is where assessment instruments are used as a guide to focus clinical assessment and decision making. Whilst assessment instruments do not replace individual assessment, they can serve as a structure and anchor to assist clinicians in their complex task of deciding who is displaying risk signs and what are the significance of these within the overall presentation. A number of assessment instruments are readily available for mental health nurses to use in their clinical practice, and although some of these have been detailed, no specific recommendations are made as to whether or not the individual mental health nurse should be using these in his or her practice. The instruments discussed have been found by the authors to be useful for clinical risk decision making, but individual services need to evaluate what meets their own clinical needs. Finally, whatever instruments mental health nurses do use to support their practice, they need to ensure they have permission to use the unaltered instruments and they have the skills, knowledge and ability to use them.

References

Alexander, L. (1999) *The Functions of Self-injury and its Link to Traumatic Events in College Students*. University of Massachusetts Amherst Dissertation, Services 9932285.

Almvik, R. & Woods, P. (1998) The Brøset Violence Checklist (BVC) and the prediction of inpatient violence: some preliminary results. *Psychiatric Care*, **5**(6), 208–211.

Babor, T.F., Higgins-Biddle, J.C., Saunders, J.B. & Monteiro, M.G. (2001) *AUDIT – The Alcohol Use Disorders Identification Test: Guidelines for Use in Primary Care*, 2nd edn. Department of Mental Health and Substance Dependence, WHO, Geneva.

Bech, P. (1994) Measurement by observations of aggressive behaviour and activities in clinical situations. *Criminal Behaviour and Mental Health*, **4**, 290–302.

Beck, A.T. & Steer, R.A. (1988) *Manual for the Beck Hopelessness Scale*. Psychological Corporation, San Antonio, Texas.

Beck, A.T. & Steer, R.A. (1991) *Manual for the Beck Scale for Suicide Ideation*. Psychological Corporation, San Antonio, Texas.

Beck, A.T., Weissman, A., Lester, D. & Trexler, L. (1974a) The measurement of pessimism: the hopelessness scale. *Journal of Clinical Psychology*, **42**, 861–865.

Beck, A.T., Schuyler, D. & Herman, J. (1974b) Development of Suicidal Intent Scales. In: *The Prediction of Suicide* (eds A.T. Beck, H. Resnick & D. Lettieri). Charles Press, Bowie, Maryland.

Bjørkly, S. (1996) Report form for aggressive episodes: preliminary report. *Percept Mot Skills*, **83**(3 Part 2), 1139–1152.

Boer, D., Hart, S., Kropp, P. & Webster, C. (1998) *Manual for the Sexual Violence Risk-20: Professional Guidelines for Assessing Risk of Sexual Violence*. Psychological Assessment Resources, Lutz, Florida.

Bowers, L., Nijman, H. & Palmstierna, T. (2007) The attempted and actual assault scale (attacks). *International Journal of Methods Psychiatric Research*, **16**(3), 171–176.

Bryman, A. & Cramer, D. (1997) *Quantitative Data Analysis with SPSS for Windows: A Guide for Social Scientists*. Routledge, London.

Cohen-Mansfield, J. (1986) Agitated behaviors in the elderly. II. Preliminary results in the cognitively deteriorated. *Journal of the American Geriatrics Society*, **34**(10), 722–727.

Cutliffe, J.R. & Barker, P. (2004) The Nurses' Global Assessment of Suicide Risk (NGASR): developing a tool for clinical practice. *Journal of Psychiatric and Mental Health Nursing*, **11**(4), 393–400.

Derogatis, L.R. (1992) *SCL-90–R: Administration, Scoring and Procedures Manual II for the Revised Version and Other Instruments of the Psychopathology Rating Scale Series*. Clinical Psychometric Research, Townson, Maryland.

Ewing, J.A. (1984) Detecting alcoholism: the CAGE questionnaire. *Journal of American Medical Association*, **252**, 1905–1907.

Finkel, S.I., Lyons, J.S. & Anderson, R.L. (1993) A brief agitation rating scale (BARS) for nursing home elderly. *Journal of the American Geriatrics Society*, **41**(1), 50–52.

Gavin, D.R., Ross, H.E. & Skinner, H.A. (1989) Diagnostic validity of the Drug Abuse Screening Test (DAST) in the assessment of DSM-III drug disorders. *British Journal of Addiction*, **84**(3), 301–307.

Hanson, R.K. (1997) *The Development of a Brief Actuarial Risk Scale for Sexual Offense Recidivism*. (User Report 97-04). Department of the Solicitor General of Canada, Ottawa.

Hanson, R. & Harris, A. (2000) *The Sex Offender Need Assessment Rating (SONAR): A Method for Measuring Change in Risk Levels*. Department of the Solicitor General of Canada, Ottawa.

Hanson, R.K. & Thornton, D. (1999) *Static-99: Improving Actuarial Risk Assessments for Sex Offenders*. User Report 99-02. Department of the Solicitor General of Canada, Ottawa.

Hanson, R. & Thornton, D. (2000) Improving risk assessments for sex offenders: a comparison of three actuarial scales. *Law & Human Behaviour*, **24**(1), 119–136.

Hare, R.D. (1991) *The Hare Psychopathy Checklist-Revised*. Multi-Health Systems, Toronto.

Hare, R.D. (2003) *Hare Psychopathy Checklist-Revised (PCL-R): 2nd Edition*. Multi-Health Systems, Toronto.

Hoffmann, N.G. & Shulman, G.D. (2005) *Avoid the Perils of 'Instrument Abuse': Good Tools Badly Used Can Harm Clients*. Highbeam Encyclopedia. Available at http://www.encyclopedia.com/doc/1G1-136563965.html (accessed 28 March 2008).

Kay, S.R., Wolkenfeld, F. & Murrill, L.M. (1988) Profiles of aggression among psychiatric patients. II. Covariates and predictors. *Journal of Nervous and Mental Disease*, **176**(9), 547–557.

Kerlinger, F.N. (1973) *Foundations of Behavioral Research*, 2nd edn. Holt Rinehart and Winston, New York.

Kropp, P. & Hart, D. (2004) *The Development of the Brief Spousal Assault Form for the Evaluation of Risk (B-SAFER): A Tool for Criminal Justice Professionals*. Department of Justice Canada, Research and Statistics Division, Ottawa.

Kropp, P.R., Hart, S.D., Webster, C.D. & Eaves, D. (1999) *Manual for the Spousal Assault Risk Assessment Guide*, 3rd edn. Multi-Health Systems, Toronto.

Moody, L.E. (1990) *Advancing Nursing Science Through Research*, Vol. 1. Sage, London.

Nijman, H.L.I., Muris, P., Merckelbach, H.L.G.J., *et al.* (1999a) The Staff Observation Aggression Scale-Revised SOAS-R. *Aggressive Behavior*, **25**(3), 197–209.

Nijman, H.L.I., Muris, P., Merckelbach, H.L.G.J., *et al.* (1999b) The Staff Observation Aggression Scale-Revised (SOAS-R): erratum. *Aggressive Behavior*, **25**(6), 476–476.

Oppenheim, A.N. (1992) *Questionnaire Design, Interviewing and Attitude Measurement*. Pinter, London.

Osuch, E.A. (undated) *Self-Injury Motivation Scale (SIMS) Version 2*. Available at http://www.centerforthestudyoftraumaticstress.org/downloads/SIMS_ver2.pdf (accessed 2 April 2008).

Osuch, E.A., Noll, J.G. & Putnam, F.W. (1999) The motivations for self-injury in psychiatric inpatients. *Psychiatry*, **62**, 334–346.

Overall, J.E. & Gorham, D.R. (1962) The Brief Psychiatric Rating Scale. *Psychological Reports*, **10**, 799–812.

Oxford University Press (1995) *The Oxford Dictionary of Current English*. Oxford University Press, Oxford.

Patel, V. & Hope, R.A. (1992) A rating scale for aggressive behaviour in the elderly: the RAGE. *Psychological Medicine*, **22**(1), 211–221.

Patterson, W., Dohn, H., Bird, J. & Patterson, G. (1983) Evaluation of suicidal patients: the SAD PERSONS Scale. *Psychosomatics*, **24**, 343–349.

Pierce, D.W. (1977) Suicidal intent in self-injury. *British Journal of Psychiatry*, **130**, 377–385.

Pierce, D.W. (1981) The predictive validation of a suicide intent scale: a five year follow-up. *British Journal of Psychiatry*, **139**, 391–396.

Polit, D.F. & Hungler, B.P. (1993) *Essentials of Nursing Research: Methods, Appraisal, and Utilization*, 3rd edn. Lippincott, Philadelphia.

Quinsey, V.L., Harris, G.T., Rice, M.E. & Cormier, C.A. (1998) *Violent Offenders: Appraising and Managing Risk*. American Psychological Association, Washington, DC.

Reed, V. & Woods, P. (2000) *The Behavioral Status Index: A Life Skills Assessment for Selecting and Monitoring Therapy in Mental Health Care*. Psychometric Press, Sheffield.

Robson, C. (1993) *Real World Research: A Resource for Social Scientists and Practitioners-Researchers*. Blackwell, Oxford.

Santa Mina, E.E., Gallop, R., Links, P., Heslegrave, R., Pringle, D., Wekerle, C. & Grewal, P. (2006) The Self-Injury Questionnaire: evaluation of the psychometric properties in a clinical population. *Journal of Psychiatric and Mental Health Nursing*, **13**(2), 221–227.

Selzer, M.L. (1971) The Michigan Alcohol Screening Test (MAST): the quest for a new diagnostic instrument. *American Journal of Psychiatry*, **127**, 1653–1658.

Spielberger, C.D. (1999) *State-Trait Anger Expression Inventory-2 (STAXI-2)*. Psychological Assessment Resources Incorporated, Odessa, Florida.

Webster, C.D., Douglas, K.S., Eaves, D. & Hart, S.D. (1997) *HCR-20: Assessing Risk for Violence. Version 2*. Mental Health, Law, and Policy Institute, Simon Fraser University, Burnaby.

Webster, C.D., Martin, M.L., Brink, J., Nicholls, T.L. & Middleton, C. (2004) *Manual for the Short Term Assessment of Risk and Treatability (START). Version 1.0, Consultation Edition.* St. Joseph's Healthcare, Hamilton, Ontario, and Forensic Psychiatric Services Commission, Port Coquitlam, British Columbia.

Wong, S.C.P. & Gordon, A.E. (2000) *Violence Risk Scale.* Research Unit, Regional Psychiatric Centre, Saskatoon, Saskatchewan.

Wong, S.C.P., Olver, M.E., Nicholaichuk, T.P. & Gordon, A.E. (2003) *Violence Risk Scale: Sexual Offenders.* Research Unit, Regional Psychiatric Centre, Saskatoon, Saskatchewan.

Yudofsky, S.C., Silver, J.M., Jackson, W., Endicott, J. & Williams, D. (1986) The Overt Aggression Scale for the objective rating of verbal and physical aggression. *American Journal of Psychiatry*, **143**, 35–39.

Chapter 5

Risk to Others

Phil Woods

Introduction

For mental health nurses an important and increasing part of their every-day practice is the assessment and management of risk to others. Steadman *et al.* (2000) state how violence risk assessment is a core feature of clinical practice in many settings from institutional to community care. However, they go on to indicate that although occurrence of these assessments is frequent, the research literature on clinical prediction is somewhat troublesome. Indeed, this area of research is an inexact science, a contentious issue and has been the focus of immense debate over the last three decades.

Anderson *et al.* (2004) indicate that there are two reasons for the focus on risk to others in clinical practice. The first is that to ignore, or fail to acknowledge, the risks to those working with patients with mental health problems leaves medical personnel unprepared. A lack of preparation leads to situations in which staff are less willing to work with aggressive patients. Finally, this will culminate in a lack of resources for those potentially most in need. Second, as society becomes more aware of what relationship does exist between mental illness and violence, risk assessments of those with mental illness will be carried out on an increasing basis in clinical, correctional and legal situations. Whilst there is some debate in the research literature as to whether or not this relationship exists, the mere fact that society thinks it does is important as clinicians may find themselves liable for failing to adequately assess and manage risk in relation to risk toward others (Bloom *et al.* 2005). Doyle and Dolan (2002, p.649) highlight that:

> *'Throughout history most societies have assumed a link between mental disorder and violence to others . . . a small number of incidents have received considerable media attention and left a strong impression of the potential dangerousness to the public of individuals with various forms of mental disorder.'*

Risk to others is fundamentally concerned with issues of violence or aggression, and is closely linked with the term dangerousness. This can involve physical, verbal, intimidating or threatening behaviours, and offending behaviour, such as assault, murder, or even arson. In fact patients with mental health problems can display a range of behaviours which involve a risk to others both inside and outside of what is deemed an offence by law. Within the vast research literature on risk to others terms such as 'violence' and 'aggression' are used so interchangeably and many different definitions have been proposed. For the purposes of this chapter, aggression, violence and risk to others will be defined as follows:

- **Aggression:** *'a disposition, a willingness to inflict harm, regardless of whether this is behaviourally or verbally expressed and regardless of whether physical harm is sustained'* (National Institute for Health and Clinical Excellence 2005, p.79).
- **Violence:** *'the use of physical force which is intended to hurt or injure another person'* (Wright *et al.* 2002a, p.7).
- **Risk to others:** *'the potential ability to cause serious physical and psychological harm to others. It also includes those fear-inducing, impulsive and destructive behaviours that are displayed or have been known to be displayed'* (Woods 2001, p.85).

This chapter raises some of the issues the mental health nurse will encounter in the assessment and management of risk to others. It cannot be totally inclusive yet tries to highlight the more important issues that readers will have to consider in relation to their own specific clinical practice areas. Many of the demographic and clinical variables, particularly the links between violence and mental health, are discussed.

How common is violence in psychiatric patients?

There has been extensive research examining this very question, prior to and during admission, as well as following discharge. Many of the earlier studies have been criticised owing to methodological flaws and consequently researchers are trying to overcome these in more recent studies.

Blumenthal and Lavender (2001, p.23) undertook a comprehensive review of the literature examining mental disorder and violence. They concluded for studies that had examined violence prior to admission that prevalence rates varied between 10 and 40%. Furthermore, data might not be that useful as violence was often reported as criteria for admission. Moreover, patients fearful of admission may react with threats and violence.

Fisher (1994) discusses how in-patient violence has always been a problem for mental health workers. Indeed, it is common in many countries. Often violence results in hospitalisation and/or disruptions to work, social, family and other commitments. Moreover, this violence causes significant problems for the treatment environment, other patients and staff (Flannery *et al.* 1994; Bensley *et al.* 1997; Morrison 1998; Owen *et al.* 1998a; Davies 2001; Needham *et al.* 2004).

Reviews have commonly shown violence to be a problem, and an ever-increasing problem. Over the last 30 years a number of reviews of psychiatric in-patient violence have been published (Haller and Deluty 1988; Drinkwater and Gudjonsson 1989; Krakowski *et al.* 1989; Mawson 1990; Aquilina 1991; Shah *et al.* 1991), largely determining that violence is common in psychiatric wards (Fottrell 1980; Tardiff and Sweillam 1982; Tardiff 1984; Pearson *et al.* 1986; Edwards *et al.* 1988; Noble and Rodger 1989; Reid *et al.* 1989; James *et al.* 1990; Miller *et al.* 1993), but the risk of serious injury is slight (Fottrell *et al.* 1978; Fottrell 1980; Pearson *et al.* 1986; Cooper and Mendonca 1991). Many of these reviews have found that most of the violence occurs against nurses (Fottrell *et al.* 1978; Fottrell 1980; Edwards *et al.* 1988; Larkin *et al.* 1988; Noble and Rodger 1989; James *et al.* 1990). Within these studies estimates of in-patient violence range considerably and are affected by base-rates and accuracy of recording.

Blumenthal and Lavender (2001, p.24) report from their comprehensive literature review that:

- the prevalence of in-patient violence varied between 10 and 40%;
- the minority of patients are responsible for most assaults;
- related factors include illness, age, substance abuse, violent history, symptom severity and situational factors such as overcrowding and nursing practices;
- nurses are the most frequent victims;
- circumstances in the settings may actually contribute to violence.

They concluded that in-patient violence rates were variable among studies and difficult to compare owing to differing patient groups, settings and definitions of violence, and therefore little could be concluded from these.

More recently, the Healthcare Commission National Audit of Violence 2006–2007 in England and Wales reported some troubling results:

- *'Findings from the audit showed that across England and Wales, in mental health services for adults of working age, levels of experienced violence were high. Many respondents reported not only a heightened frequency of incidents, but also an increased severity – in extreme cases involving weapons'* (The

Audit Team, Royal College of Psychiatrists' Centre for Quality Improvement 2007a, p.13).

- *'The audit found that 64% of nurses on older people's wards reported that they had been physically assaulted'* (The Audit Team, Royal College of Psychiatrists' Centre for Quality Improvement 2007b, p.2).

Public perception still exists that those with a mental illness, especially psychosis, when discharged to the community will be a danger to others. Some people with a mental illness will be violent, but many are not. Whilst the issue has been extensively studied, one landmark study and three recent studies are reported below to allow the reader to get a sense of this.

Johnnie Baxstrom was sentenced to imprisonment for assault in 1959. In 1966 he was transferred to the Dannemora State Hospital for the criminally insane, where he was detained beyond his sentence expiry date. The Supreme Court in the USA upheld his appeal that his constitutional rights had been violated. Baxstrom was released and this led to the release of 966 individuals from maximum security hospitals to lower security institutions or into the community. Steadman and Cocozza (1974) followed this group up for a period of 4 years, finding that only 20% had been reconvicted, predominantly for non-violent offences, calling into question the accuracy of dangerousness predictions that had previously been made. Furthermore, this also indicates that few were actually a risk to others whilst living in the community.

Blumenthal and Lavender (2001, p.26) report how early studies concluded that psychiatric patients were no more likely to be violent than the general population. However, much of this research took place when policy meant that the most seriously mentally ill were confined to in-patient care. As policy changed more to deinstitutionalisation, studies started to find patients were more likely to be arrested or convicted for violent offences. Furthermore, many methodological flaws have made interpretation difficult.

The largest study of late to examine how common violence is in the community was the MacArthur study on mental disorder (Monahan *et al.* 2001). The researchers recruited 1,136 patients into the study and followed them up 12 months post-discharge. Although over the course of the study attrition was high, some interesting results emerged. Approximately 25% of the patients reported a violent incident (not including verbal aggression) and about 50% of these patients reported more than one violent incident during the follow-up period. The researchers also reported that this did not mean that those discharged were more risky to others than their community neighbours. It was more likely that such variables as substance abuse were a contributory factor as once this was controlled they were no more likely than their neighbours to be violent.

The Five Year Report of the National Confidential Inquiry into Suicide and Homicide by People with Mental Illness (Appleby *et al.* 2006) reported that there were 2,684 homicides in England and Wales between April 1999 and December 2003. Of these, 261 (10%) were described in psychiatric reports as having mental illness at the time of the offence. The report highlights that 249 had contact with mental health services within the last 12 months and from these, 15 were in-patients at the time of offence and in 43 cases the offence took place within 3 months of their discharge. Data translate into 52 patient homicides per year and rates are reported to be neither rising nor falling from previous inquires. The report does indicate whether some of these homicides were considered preventable.

In summary, violence is certainly a problem for in-patient mental health settings. This is perhaps not surprising considering that nowadays it is mostly more acute and complex patients that find themselves admitted to hospital when community treatment is not appropriate. On the other hand violence in the community is not as high as perhaps the media would want the public to believe. However, the problem does exist and it could be more of a problem, and perhaps a more preventable one, than some clinicians may realise.

Violence prediction

It follows on that if violence is such a frequently occurring phenomenon in mental health practice then how can it be predicted so it is known who is going to be violent and who is not? It is probably fair to say that traditionally violence prediction has been a difficult clinical task, with very mixed results and different priorities in different areas of practice. In all areas of practice, short- and medium-term prediction and the identification of associated variables are very important, yet in areas such as forensic psychiatry long-term prediction is also a very key issue and is highly associated with the patient's offending behaviour. Research using statistical approaches has at times been able to discriminate between the violent and the not violent, yet only with moderate accuracy. Moreover, studies over shorter periods of time tend to achieve greater accuracy.

In a seminal paper, Monahan (1981) reviewed the 'first generation' of violence prediction research, much of which relied solely on professional judgement in relation to the probability of future violence. He concluded that the 'best' clinical research in existence at the time indicated that psychiatrists and psychologists were accurate in no more than one out of three predictions of violent behaviour. Although it appears that clinicians' predictions were worse-than-chance, it has been later explained that it more reflected an overcautiousness on the part of professionals who (without the benefit of empirical data) opted to err on the side of caution (Rice *et al.* 2002).

Later studies have reported that psychiatrists, in particular, tend to overpredict future violence; however, they are better at predicting violence in the acute setting or from patients suffering from an acute psychiatric illness (Johnson 2000). Moreover, when the risk factors are outlined and the patient's current situation is understood, psychiatrists have only been able to predict aggression with moderate accuracy in the short term (Johnson 2000). Thus, there appear to be real problems with accurately predicting violence in psychiatric patients, and some have argued this is because the necessary tools are missing to enhance the task (Monahan 1984; McNiel and Binder 1994; Rabinowitz and Garelik-Wyler 1999; Soliman and Reza 2001).

More recently, studies have reported improved accuracy from clinicians (Hoptman *et al.* 1999; Grove *et al.* 2000; Lewis and Webster 2004; Norko and Baranoski 2005), but research is ongoing to try to improve the issue more through structured clinical judgement approaches.

Approaches to the assessment of risk to others

As discussed above, most assessment of risk to others has developed around violence and aggression. Over many decades now the violence risk assessment literature has focused on patient clinical, contextual and historical factors empirically associated with aggression, and on the accuracy of clinicians in predicting aggression (Borum 1996). Historically, two main approaches have developed to assist in the assessment and related management of risk to others; and this is perhaps owing to the fact that clinicians and researchers have approached violence risk assessment from very different perspectives. Clinicians have tended to assess the risk of violence using unaided clinical judgement, whilst researchers have seemed to focus on risk prediction in large, heterogeneous populations, employing relatively static actuarial predictors (Borum 1996). Over the years three clear iterations in relation to these approaches have emerged.

The first approach to the assessment of risk to others is the *clinical* approach, which is based on professional opinion concerning a patient's self-presentation and on consideration of clinical or situational variables. Of course this opinion depends on the clinician's skill, knowledge and experience (Anderson *et al.* 2004). This approach looks for explanations of specific violent behaviour and is concerned with:

- how individuals behave;
- how they react in various situations;

- how they have been known to behave;
- how willingly they accept treatment;
- how much insight they have into their condition.

Many have opposed the clinical approach on the grounds that it may be contaminated by assessor bias, and it is only as good as its theoretical base. Others have indicated how it has demonstrated low inter-rater reliability, low validity and failed to specify the decision-making process (Monahan and Steadman 1994), and low predictive validity compared to actuarial predictions (Lidz *et al.* 1993; Mossman 1994). Further evidence that has been used to criticise this approach is that on occasion predictions from clinicians are no better than chance (Monahan 1988); however, evidence is changing in relation to this and recent results from studies do indicate more reliable results (Grove *et al.* 2000; Lewis and Webster 2004; Norko and Baranoski 2005). Despite all of these arguments against the clinical approach it is still widely used in mental health practice today. Perhaps one of the reasons is that, as Snowden (1997) points out, its strengths lie in its flexibility and potential for violence prevention. This is a position also shared by others in that it has the advantage of being flexible, allowing for case-specific influences and violence prevention (Hart 1998, cited in Doyle and Dolan 2002, p.650).

The second approach is the *actuarial or statistical* approach. This seeks to assess the individual on predetermined, often historical, variables that have been shown to be predictive of risk to others. It is based on the assumption that an individual coming from a population within which a certain type of behaviour is common is more likely to display this form of behaviour (Doyle and Dolan 2002). In other words, actuarial decisions about risk are made according to rules and focus on risk factors that are believed to predict violence across settings and individuals (Dolan and Doyle 2000). Risk assessment tools are created using variables that have been empirically demonstrated to be predictive of risk to others.

Although actuarial approaches have consistently been shown to improve the consistency of risk assessment (Borum *et al.* 1993), there are arguments in the literature (see, for instance, Rice *et al.* 2002) that clinical factors may also be useful in the prediction of risk to others.

Currently, a strong consensus in the research literature has emerged that actuarial factors should serve as an anchor for more dynamic clinical risk assessment, and in the author's opinion quite rightly so. This is termed the third generation *structured clinical judgement* (MacLean 2000; Doyle and Dolan 2002). Webster *et al.* (1997) believe that structured clinical judgement represents an effective blend of empirical knowledge and clinical expertise. Hart (1998) agrees that some of the structured clinical instruments that have developed to support this approach promote the systematic collection of empirically grounded evidence, and unlike strict actuarial measures, they allow for flexibility and professional discretion, and take dynamic variables into consideration in the assessment of risk. Researchers are starting to examine the contribution of these dynamic risk factors (e.g. Boer *et al.* 1997; Dempster and Hart 2002) and results are suggesting that risk assessments that consider dynamic variables can be more accurate than those that rely on static variables alone. Rice *et al.* (2002) believe that '*the role of dynamic characteristics in violence risk assessment has become complicated and confused*' (p.591). They also warn that measuring any variable at only one point in time essentially makes it static.

What variables are associated with risk to others?

There is extensive literature on variables that are thought to be associated with risk to others, and a number of literature reviews have been published to summarise the evidence to date. Most of these reviews in some way or another discuss issues in relation to patient, staff and environmental factors. For example, in an extremely useful study, Johnson (2004) reviews:

- patient-related variables;
- staff-related variables (demographics, experience, satisfaction);
- unit-related variables (time of day, incident location, staffing, census, patient mix);
- interactional variables (staff–patient interactions, staff–patient rapport and coercive interactional style).

In a similar review, Anderson *et al.* (2004) organised data in relation to patient-related risk factors:

- dispositional (demographic, cognitive, personality);
- contextual (stress perception, social support, means for violence);
- clinical (diagnosis and symptom patterns, functioning, substance abuse);
- historical (prior hospitalisation and outcome, prior violence, social factors).

Whilst some comments and findings from these reviews and other literature are reported in the text that follows, the reader is directed towards these to obtain more detail on the relationships. Below some of the patient-related variables in relation to risk to others will be briefly discussed.

Patient-related variables

Patient gender

There is certainly a lay understanding that male gender is more associated with risk to others, especially young men. Whilst it is probably true that males commit more violent crimes towards others, and in the general population males are more prone to violence than females and the violence is more severe and more likely to cause harm (Otto 2000), it does not appear to hold true in all studies that males are more likely to be risky to others in the psychiatric setting.

Wright *et al.* (2002a, p.19) state that *'studies of in-patient populations consistently conclude that male patients do not necessarily pose greater risk than female patients, although this is not unanimous'*. Monahan *et al.* (2001, p.43) conclude on the MacArthur study on mental disorder and violence that *'men are no more likely to be violent than women over the course of the 1 year follow-up period'*; however, *'violence committed by men is more likely to result in serious injury'*. Anderson *et al.* (2004) suggest, based on these inconsistencies in the literature, caution in the use of gender as a baseline risk factor for violence.

Age

Age is one of the most commonly studied patient-related variables in relation to its association with risk to others; however, the literature is full of inconsistent results (Johnson 2004). Wright *et al.* (2002a, p.20) summarise how studies do not agree up to what age a higher risk exists, but that most studies agree that risk of violence does decrease with age. It also seems that there is an interaction effect between age and gender and risk to others. Anderson *et al.* (2004) indicate that in the general population, age is a well-known risk factor for violence and criminal behaviour, and that it holds true for the mentally ill as well. Nonetheless, they also state that, as with all risk factors for violence, age must be considered in the light of contextual factors such as mental state and the patient environment.

Ethnicity

Wright *et al.* (2002a, p.20) report how *'research findings concerning ethnicity and dangerousness in psychiatric patients are both controversial and highly confounded by intervening variables'* and this is perhaps the most important thing to bear in mind in the relationship between ethnicity and risk to others. Furthermore, Johnson (2004) concludes that ethnicity has not been shown to be a significant factor in in-patient aggression. Anderson *et al.* (2004) suggest that while rates of violent behaviour are thought to differ across racial lines, these are highly related to contextual risk factors.

Diagnosis

The relationship between diagnosis (or mental disorder/mental illness) and risk to others is probably one of the most controversial areas in relation to risk assessment. The press (and the public in some instances) would perhaps have us believe there is a strong association, particularly when one or two extreme cases are given high-profile press coverage. However, the fact remains that the majority of those with a mental disorder do not pose a significant risk to others at all. Not surprisingly the research literature is also not that helpful and for each study that finds some association with risk to others there is another that finds it to be a protective factor. However, there are some indications of potential risk factors that need to be considered that emerge from this literature. For instance, certain symptoms of psychotic disorders, personality disorder (particularly antisocial and borderline) and psychopathy appear to be significant risk factors.

In a landmark study that tried to examine the relationship between mental disorder and violence Swanson *et al.* (1990) administered the Diagnostic Interview Schedule (DIS) to a representative sample of community dwelling adults who were part of the Epidemiologic Catchment Area (ECA) survey. Their main findings were that individuals who met DIS criteria for a psychiatric disorder were more likely to engage in violent behaviour than participants who did not meet those criteria. The highest rates of violence were found among those who also reported substance abuse and young men aged 18–24 years in the lowest socioeconomic group. The increased relative risk of violence in psychotic disorders found in this study also suggested that there was some factor specific to psychotic disorders that was responsible for the higher relative risk (Wright *et al.* 2002a), and consequently this prompted research to be undertaken into specific symptoms.

Researchers have studied the association between delusions and violence. Whilst many have reported an association (Häfner and Böker 1982; Taylor 1985; Taylor *et al.* 1994, 1998; Buchanan 1997) there are others that have not (e.g. Junginger *et al.* 1998).

Command hallucinations have also been studied, as generally such symptoms are considered to be a potential predictive factor of risk to others. Results have not always supported the association (Hellerstein *et al.* 1987; Junginger 1995; Kaspar *et al.* 1996) although patients do report complying with the commands in some of the studies. Rudnick (1999) has undertaken a review on the subject and, based on the literature to that date, concluded that studies indicated no link between command hallucinations and violence. However, this does not mean that a relationship does not exist and more research is needed.

Threat-control override (TCO) symptoms are the belief that one's internal controls are being overridden by an external force (e.g. delusions of passivity, thought insertion and persecutory delusions). Link and Stueve (1994) were probably the first to note that these TCO symptoms created an increased risk of violence independent of other symptoms of psychosis and other studies have found similar results (Swanson *et al.* 1996, 1997; Link *et al.* 1998). However, Appelbaum *et al.* (2000) and Monahan *et al.* (2001) reporting data from the MacArthur study on mental disorder and violence found that neither delusions nor TCO symptoms were associated with higher risk of violence in the year after discharge from hospital. Indeed, Mullen (1997) and Stompe *et al.* (2004) have questioned the original concept itself. This calls for researchers to examine TCO symptoms more fully in future work.

Although results in relation to delusions, command hallucinations and TCO symptoms are not conclusive yet, generally researchers still feel all three symptom groups have a significant role to play in risk to others. Therefore, clinicians need to consider these in relation to the overall mental state of the patient and how these relate to other significant risk factors.

Prior history of violence

A prior history of violence, particularly if it is recent in nature, is one of the most important and consistently associated patient-related historical risk factors for in-patient violence (Anderson *et al.* 2004; Johnson 2004). In fact, a number of authors have previously observed that a prior history of violence is the most consistent predictor of in-patient violence (Aiken 1984; McNiel *et al.* 1988; Noble and Rodger 1989; Blomhoff *et al.* 1990; Owen *et al.* 1998b; Soliman and Reza 2001).

Substance abuse

Within the literature one of the most striking themes is how substance abuse has been found to be one of the most reliable risk factors that contribute to risk to others (e.g. Swanson *et al.* 1990, 1996; Dittmann 1996; Fulwiler *et al.* 1997; Phillips 2000; Soyka 2000; Steadman *et al.* 2000; Steinert 2001; Wright *et al.* 2002b; D'Silva and Ferriter 2003; Norko and Baranoski 2005). For instance, Wallace *et al.* (2004) found a significant association between schizophrenia and criminal convictions, with substance abuse increasing the likelihood 16-fold. Similarly, Cuffel *et al.* (1994) studied those individuals diagnosed with schizophrenia or schizoaffective disorder to determine whether substance abuse increased the risk for violence. The results demonstrated that use of drugs and/or alcohol was associated with increases in concurrent and future violent behaviour when compared with persons with schizophrenia and no substance use. Violence was particularly elevated for individuals having a pattern of polysubstance use involving illicit substances. Therefore, substance abuse needs to be considered in any assessment of risk to others.

This section has just touched on some of the variables that have been associated with risk to others. Many other variables have not been examined. Whilst the author does not wish to downplay their importance in the overall picture of risk to others, the extent and focus of this chapter does not allow for extensive examination of these. The reader is directed to the reviews cited if interested in the findings relative to the very many variables that have been researched.

Woods and Lasiuk (2008, p.7), summarising their literature review on risk prediction, state how:

'... several trends are apparent from the literature reviewed. The first is that violence correlates significantly with sociodemographic (i.e., criminal history, male gender, age, low income, low education, etc.), environmental factors, and to some extent mental disorder. The evidence concerning the relationship between psychosis and violence, although somewhat mixed, seems to indicate that suspiciousness, hostility, agitation-excitement, and thinking disturbance are most often associated with violence. It is clear that substance abuse is a consistent risk factor for violence, both on its own and combined with mental disorder'.

Assessing risk to others

This section was written with the mental health nurse in mind and suggestions are considered in relation to this. However, mental health nurses work as part of multidisciplinary teams, and ideally risk decisions should be made within these teams. As Doyle and Dolan (2002, p.650) point out:

'... mental health nurses are a major source of clinical information that needs to be considered by the nurse and the team as a whole when assessing risks ... have access to 24-h observation of behaviour and greater opportunities than other professionals to develop relationships ... are constantly making decisions on the level of risk.... This unique position makes the role of the mental health nurse crucial to the process of assessing and managing violence risk'.

Therefore, this should be considered when reading the following suggestions in relation to risk assessment and management of harm to others.

Consider the four different scenarios in Box 5.1:

- What is different about them?
- How would you go about assessing risk to others differently?
- Should you do things differently?
- Who is the highest risk?

Box 5.1   Four risk scenarios for Jack.

Scenario one

Jack, a known offender, is admitted to your ward. He has a long history of assaults on others and has served many periods of time in prison and on forensic units as a result of these. He is currently very psychotic and is expressing thoughts of harming others.

Scenario two

Jack is admitted to your ward in a very psychotic state. He is expressing thoughts of harming others. However, Jack is well known to the service and has expressed these thoughts before but has never carried them out.

Scenario three

Jack is admitted to your ward in a very psychotic state. He is expressing thoughts of harming others. Jack is unknown to the service.

Scenario four

Jack is admitted to your ward in a very psychotic state. He is not expressing any thoughts of harming others. Jack is unknown to the service.

These are perhaps some of the questions that may come into your mind.

Clearly there are historical data available for scenarios one and two, but for scenarios three and four, history is unknown. So should this make a difference? In a previous section it was indicated that history of violence is a good predictor of violence in the future. However, should you use historical data for scenario two and Jack's self-report in scenario four? The plain and simple answer is the mental health nurse should treat all four scenarios equally and do an assessment of risk to others for Jack; otherwise he/she may miss some potential risk factor, resulting in someone being harmed. The point that is being made is that all patients when admitted should undergo an assessment of risk to others if assessment is to be done effectively.

It is clear from discussion previously in this chapter and Chapters 2 and 3 of this book that structured clinical judgement is the way forward for mental health nurses in their assessment of risk to others. Some of the tools that can be used to assist the assessment of risk to others have been discussed in Chapter 4. This chapter's author urges mental health nurses to utilise one or more of these to assist in structured assessment of risk to others. However, these will not give them all the answers and clinical assessments will also need to be undertaken.

Many frameworks have been developed to help mental health nurses and other professionals focus their assessments of risk. Box 5.2 summarises some of the recent suggestions outlined by the Department of Health (2007).

Box 5.2 Risk factors for violence (Department of Health 2007, pp. 51–52).

Demographic factors:

- male
- young age
- socially disadvantaged neighbourhoods
- lack of social support
- employment problems
- criminal peer group

Background history:

- childhood maltreatment
- history of violence
- first violent at young age
- history of childhood conduct disorder
- history of non-violent criminality

Clinical history:

- psychopathy
- substance abuse
- personality disorder
- schizophrenia
- executive dysfunction
- non-compliance with treatment

Psychological and psychosocial factors:

- anger
- impulsivity
- suspiciousness
- morbid jealously
- criminal/violent attitudes
- command hallucinations
- lack of insight

Current context:

- threats of violence
- interpersonal discord/instability
- availability of weapons

Wellman (2006, pp.57–159), when discussing questioning approaches to assess risk to others (particularly violence), suggests the following are asked:

- *'how the patient experiences and copes with frustration and anger*
- *their involvement in fights and other forms of violence both as a juvenile and as an adult*

- *their involvement in any violent gangs or subcultures*
- *any history of emotional, verbal or physical abuse of partners, family members or children*
- *any history of sexual aggression or offending*
- *any arrests, criminal record or unconvicted involvement in violent offending*
- *any episodes of indiscriminate verbal or physical hostility*
- *any history of violence to health or social care staff*
- *any history of damage to property, or arson*
- *any history of violence driven by hallucinations or delusions'*

Furthermore, Wellman highlights assessing intent following any violent behaviour as a useful mechanism to determine:

- antecedents (circumstantial factors, provocation, intoxication, treatment status);
- behaviour (planned or impulsive, directed and specific to one person, weapon use, interventions used); and
- consequences (degree of harm or damage caused, victim empathy, positive reinforcers, perception of violent behaviour).

Morgan and Wetherell (2004) indicate how it is important to place the risk assessment in relation to the context (e.g. changing personal circumstances, may be risky in one situation but not another) and the environment (e.g. how well functioning, current environment and community in which the patient lives, local hazards, emotional arousal, potential weapons), as well as to call on research information. Daffern and Howells (2002, p.479) suggest:

'. . . a distinction can be made between structural assessment approaches, which emphasise the correct classification of the form of a particular behaviour, and functional assessment approaches, which emphasise the purpose of the behaviour'.

Some issues that need to be considered in the assessment of risk to others

The following are some of the issues that the mental health nurse should consider in the assessment of risk to others. These are presented in no particular order as each is highly overlapping with each of the others. It is not intended to be a comprehensive list and consideration also needs to be given to the factors that have been discussed above which have emerged from the research into risk to others (for example, the demographic and situational variables). Again it is highlighted that nurses where possible should utilise one or more of the instruments that are available to assist with the assessment of risk to others.

Verbal aggression and threatening behaviour

Verbal aggression and threatening behaviour can occur for a number of reasons and can have a major impact on the individual who is on the receiving end of this. It is important to assess this fully as it can be a precursor to some other form of violent behaviour; or it can be a means to an end in itself. Sometimes the threat of an attack can be more stressful than the attack itself. It can also be the way someone reacts when angry.

Assessment should include the severity and frequency of the verbal aggression or threats. It is useful to utilise some form of charting to collect this sort of information in a systematic and structured way. Many instruments exist that can help in the process and some of these are discussed in Chapter 4 of this book. Hospital incident reporting systems may also contain relevant data. When information is available on past verbal aggression and threatening behaviour this will allow current behaviour to be placed within the context of historical data. For both current and historical data it is vital to determine if any trigger events exist that are a precursor to this behaviour or does it just occur totally out of the blue and for no apparent reason? Other information that should be collected in relation to past and present behaviour is:

- Did the patient target any particular person or could the verbal aggression have been directed towards anyone?
- Does this verbal aggression usually escalate into other forms of behaviour?
- What interventions have worked in the past?

Stalking should also be considered – the more obvious form of physical stalking as well as methods such as the internet, cell/mobile phone texting, telephone and letter. This stalking may be obvious when a particular person is being targeted, but at other times it may be very difficult to find out about. Stalking may also be related to sexually threatening behaviour.

Often there is a tendency to under-report verbal aggression and threatening behaviour in clinical practice. Whilst this occurs for a number of reasons it needs to be borne in mind during the assessment. If a patient is frequently verbally aggressive sometimes staff tolerate this as normal behaviour for the person. Therefore, in some cases mental health nurses may need to consider that the extent of previous verbal aggression and threatening behaviour may be vastly underestimated by their current assessment.

Previous violence towards others

This is probably one of the most important and foremost parts of the assessment the mental health nurse will undertake if a patient is threatening harm to someone else, as one of the greatest predictive factors of the risk to others is when violence has occurred in the past.

The severity and frequency of any violence that has occurred in the past should be assessed where information is available. Hospital incident reporting systems, police and court records may be a good source of information. Relatives or significant others and patients themselves are of course other sources. However, it should be remembered that documented evidence may be more reliable as patients and their relatives or significant others may wish to hide a previous history of violence for many reasons.

The importance of collected information on historical data about violence towards others is that it allows the mental health nurse to consider this information alongside the potential risk that has been identified during the assessment. Similar information that was important for verbal aggression and threatening behaviour is also useful to collect here. For instance:

- Were there any trigger events, or was the violence or aggression totally out of the blue and for no apparent reason?
- Did the patient target any particular person or could the attack have been directed towards anyone?
- Were weapons used and if so what?
- How was the attack stopped and what injures occurred as a result of this?
- How is all this linked to any verbal aggression or threatening behaviour that is currently occurring?
- Was the violence of a sexual nature?
- Was it a result of stalking?

These are just some of the questions that come to mind.

Mental state

Obviously mental state can have a profound effect on how risky a patient is to others. It is important to consider the results of the mental status assessment, particularly any delusions or hallucinations that are being experienced. If the patient is guarded, suspicious or paranoid, this may be a key indicator. In order to place these in the context of the assessment of overall risk to others, it is important that full details of these are explored with the patient and any significant others. It is also vital to explore the effect these are having on the patient's coping responses. Historical data will be vital if available to determine how the patient responded to similar symptoms in the past.

Insight and coping strategies

Whilst level of insight or awareness of illness or symptoms is always important, so is insight into the risk the patient is to others, or has been in the past. This gives the mental health nurse a good understanding of the view the patient has in relation to this. If the patient is indifferent to this risk this obviously has different management implications than if the patient wants to work towards reducing this risk. Awareness of tension and how the patient describes and tries to reduce this may have implications here. Also issues around stress and anger may be relevant. Does the patient feel justified in his or her feelings and lack victim or potential victim empathy? Questions such as this are all important.

Substance abuse

It is clear in the above discussion that substance abuse is significantly related to many aspects of risk to others. Whilst assessment of this is vitally important, Chapter 7 deals with this and readers are directed towards this chapter to assist in their assessment.

Offending behaviour

Particularly important for those mental health nurses that work in forensic services, but becoming more and more important for those who also work in acute or community services, is the relationship that previous offending behaviour has on risk to others. Whilst some patients may have been hospitalised because of an offence, others may have offences in their histories. Sexual offending, assault, battery, homicide and arson are all offences that come easily to mind when thinking of future risk to others. Some offences may be one-off and may never occur again, while other patients may have criminal careers. Therefore, recidivism needs to be a consideration in both the assessment process and later risk management.

Potential victim

It could be clear when a patient is presenting with a risk to others who the likely victim is. In other cases it could be anyone or unknown. Mental health nurses need to examine this issue in their overall assessment. Indicators may be previous victims or a person may come forward to express concerns. Victim availability is an important issue to consider as well as the means by which the patient has to access the potential victim.

Exploitation of vulnerability

Some patients will exploit more vulnerable people for various reasons: personal gain, sexual favours, money – to name a few ways this can occur. Sometimes this may be through bullying, fear-inducing behaviour or threats of violence to the person or significant others. Therefore, during the assessment of risk to others the mental health nurse needs to take into account these issues. The sort of information that should be collected or may be useful will be similar to that found in the sections on verbal aggression and threatening behaviour and previous violence to others.

Distinctions between short- and long-term prediction of risk to others

Within any assessment of risk of harm to others the mental health nurse is contributing towards a prediction of how likely the event will occur. Often risk assessments are placed within the context of short- and long-term risks. Some patients may only have potential short-term risks whilst their mental state is stabilised or interpersonal circumstances are resolved. Other patients will be considered to be risky to others for many years, or even the rest of their lives. For example, some sexual offenders may always be risky in certain circumstances. When undertaking an assessment of risk to others it is therefore important for mental health nurses to consider just what time scale it is in relation to. It will affect the assessment data they collect, the instruments they may utilise and the management plans that are considered.

The above are some of the main areas the mental health nurse should examine when assessing for risk to others. Behavioural observation will be a key vehicle during this assessment process. Another vehicle will be the interpersonal relationship that the nurse has with the patient. Box 5.3 summarises some of the factors that have been discussed and should be considered by mental health nurses in their assessment of risk to others.

There is no crystal ball that will help mental health nurses predict who is going to be risky to others. It is only assessment data that will provide indicators if this is a potential risk for those they work with, thus allowing related risk management plans to be implemented. Some patients may hide their risk to others during the assessment process, whilst others may openly, and sometimes proudly, tell you who is at risk from them and why. Morgan and Wetherell (2004, pp.221–222) give some good insight into the assessment of risk to others:

> *'There is no mystique about risk assessment, as with all other types of assessment it depends on the accessibility and quality of information gathered. To this end, it requires persistence in pursuit of the relevant information held at multiple sources. The skill lies more in the delicate manner and approach to enquiring after appropriate information from the service user, and all other relevant knowledge to contribute.'*

Before leaving this section on assessment, the concept of relational security needs to be briefly mentioned, especially for those mental health nurses that work in forensic areas, as this is where this concept is more prominent. According to Collins and Davies (2005), relational security is complex and:

> *'. . . in general refers to a detailed understanding of those receiving secure care and how to manage them. For example, a competent forensic nurse will have an*

Box 5.3   Summary of some factors regarding risk to others that need to be considered.

- Current behaviour (particularly verbal aggression or threats)
- Current mental state
- Has verbal aggression occurred in the past?
- Has physical aggression occurred in the past?
- Was this serious or minor?
- Were there any clear triggers?
- What was the apparent reason?
- Was there any provocation?
- What were the severity, frequency and latency?
- Who was the victim?
- Was the victim targeted or random?
- Was a weapon involved?
- Were there any accomplices?
- What was the time and location of the incident?
- How did mental state contribute to the aggression?
- Developing patterns of aggression
- Insight into actions
- Empathy for victim
- Communication skills
- Interpersonal difficulties
- Cognitive disability or distortions
- Availability of victims or weapons
- Support available from others
- What protective factors exist

extensive knowledge of a patient. This will include potential risk behaviors and a relationship with the patient that includes an open acknowledgement of the potential for dangerous behavior. This level of knowledge allows the practitioner to constantly assess behaviors, patterns of behavior and changes in mental state that have a direct relationship to any immediate or potentially dangerous behavior or similarity to offending patterns. This level of knowledge can enable care to be delivered in an environment where levels of restriction and supervision can be varied according to the needs of the patient while maintaining the protection of others' (p.41).

This is just how risk assessment should be approached in all areas of practice: constantly taking into account all related variables and adapting management plans accordingly.

Management of risk to others

Risk management is essentially the next stage following risk assessment and is an important part of the mental health nurses' practice, where they need to utilise their knowledge and skills from many areas of mental health nursing practice. Doyle (1999, p.41) has defined risk management as '*the systematic, organised effort to eliminate or reduce the likelihood of misfortune, harm, damage or loss*'. Morgan (2000, p.2) defines risk management as:

> '. . . *a statement of plans and an allocation of individual responsibilities for translating collective decisions into actions. This process should name all relevant people involved in the treatment and support including the service user and appropriate informal carers. It should also identify a review date for the assessment and management plan*'.

A number of key issues need to be considered in risk management measures that are utilised in relation to risk to others. To effectively operationalise a risk management plan mental health nurses need to state precisely and specifically the nature or level of the risk, placing this in situational context and outlining the relationships between the risky behaviours presented. Clear statements of anticipated risk and how these are, or can be, avoided need to be made; thus the impact of any risk is minimised. Early warning signs are a useful way to conceptualise the risk so it can be more easily anticipated. The risk management plan should focus specifically on the responses required to deal with any crisis that may arise (e.g. the risk is observed to occur).

It is very important that the patient is informed of the risk(s) that have been identified, what will happen if they occur and why. This could involve the individual being given the opportunity to select from a range of alternative management strategies. If this is to occur therapeutically to allow the individual to develop and hopefully learn from a risky situation, thus reducing potential risk, creative thinking that promotes positive risk-taking would need to happen (Woods 2001). Morgan and Wetherell (2004, p.216), discussing positive risk-taking, state that:

> '. . . *individuals can only grow through measured and justifiable risk-taking. . . . Life consists of exercising one choice over another, and this liberty should apply to service users as much as it does to other members of society*'.

Whilst allowing patients to enter into risky situations where someone is likely to get hurt is not being condoned here, it is more about engaging patients in conscious decisions about how they will manage their risks. Indeed, as Morgan and Wetherell (2004) further suggest, this is not a new way of working for mental health nurses as they have been engaging clients in their care for years, but maybe not so actively in relation to their risk-taking. Furthermore, Morgan and Wetherell indicate that this positive risk-taking needs to be clearly reasoned for, documented, defensible and have contingency plans in place if things go wrong, insomuch as it may face opposition and scrutiny and therefore needs to be, as Wetherell (2001) states:

- justifiable;
- measured;
- intelligent;
- negotiated with the patient and any carers.

Morgan and Hemming (1999) discuss how risk management interventions can be considered at three levels:

1. preventative (attention to working relationship, education, relapse early warning signs);
2. management of escalating situations (de-escalation, rapid response, crisis intervention);
3. post-incident support (positive support for victims, culture of learning rather than blaming).

Harris and Rice (1997) imply there are six risk management interventions:

1. static (locked doors, seclusion);
2. dynamic (restraint, electronic tagging);
3. situational (restriction of access to means or victim);
4. pharmacological;
5. interpersonal (communication and interpersonal relationship);
6. self-control (psychotherapeutic or psychosocial means).

As with any other process, the risk management needs to be continuously reviewed, within identified time constraints, with results communicated to all relevant people involved in the care process. Doyle (1999) offers some practical advice in the form of a six-stage risk management cycle:

1. identification;
2. risk assessment;
3. rating risk;
4. implement risk management measures;
5. monitoring of risk management measures;
6. risk assessment review.

He further highlights how it is easily incorporated in the care programme approach. More recently, Doyle has reported a Five-step Structured Profes-sional Approach to Risk Management (Doyle and Duffy 2006, p.146) and this can be a useful process for the mental health nurse to use in relation to risk to others:

1. case information (history, mental state, substance use);
2. presence of risk factors (historical, current, contextual);
3. presence of protective factors (historical, current, contextual);
4. risk formulation (nature, severity, imminence, likelihood, risk reducing/ enhancing);
5. management plan (treatment, management, monitoring, supervision, victim safety planning).

Discussion

Mental health nurses probably do not need to do a comprehensive assess-ment of risk to others for all patients, yet all patients should at least be screened for this risk. Some patients may present with obvious signs of risk to others, whilst others may hide the risk during the assessment. Consequently, at times things will go wrong and errors will occur. Whilst not all of these can be eliminated, two important areas may help the mental health nurse to reduce these: use of the nurse–patient relation-ship, and improving practice in the assessment and management of risk to others.

Use of the nurse–patient relationship

The use of the nurse–patient relationship is an important skill for mental health nurses to use in the assessment and management of risk to others. Indeed, it is probably the most useful tool they have available and plays a vital part in ensuring the risk management plan is effective. Kettles (2004) highlights this in her work on defining the concept of forensic risk and identifies such key skills as active listening and developing rapport as well as observation of non-verbal cues as important when interviewing during risk assessment and intervening through risk management plans. Wellman (2006) indicates that mental health nurses need to employ sensit-ivity and a non-judgemental approach. He also discusses how they need to be supportive and empathetic through the use of active listening and open-ended questions and be ready to intervene should the patient cause any distress.

Improving practice in the assessment and management of risk to others

A statement made by Borum (1996) that the extent and adequacy of the training mental health professionals receive in violence risk prediction is unclear is perhaps still somewhat true today. Whilst training is readily available to deal with violence when it actually occurs, how many mental health nurses have had training to help them in their assessment and management of risk to others outside of their basic professional training? In the author's experience, perhaps not as many as should have been trained, considering that these assessment processes and management issues are daily practice for them. According to Monahan (1993), there are four aspects to the professional prediction of risk:

1. The health professional must be instructed as to information to collect.
2. The information must be gathered.
3. The information must be used to assess risk.
4. The health professional must communicate the risk assessment to other members of the health team and to those responsible for making or implementing final clinical decisions.

This chapter author would suggest this could be a bare minimum of in-service education for every mental health nurse that is involved in the assessment of risk to others.

Some other key researchers have made some interesting recommendations for improving practice in risk assessment and management. Pollock and Webster (1990) and Monahan and Steadman (1994) highlight the importance of risk assessments being systematic and based on the population undergoing assessment; also, identified risk factors should be broken down into more manageable components, further assessed through effective treatment planning, and outcomes evaluated through recovery status. Borum (1996) promotes three recommendations to improve clinical practice in risk assessment that are still pertinent today:

1. Improve assessment technology.
2. Develop clinical practice guidelines.
3. Develop training programmes and curricula.

Bloom *et al.* (2005) suggest a number of principles that can be considered when conducting risk assessments:

- Assessments should be in line with pertinent legal tests and professional standards.
- Assessment conditions must be satisfactory and evaluated thoroughly.

- Assessment must be specific to the risk issue being considered.
- Assessing for risk of violence is broader than predicting it.
- Actuarial information obtained from records can focus and strengthen assessments.
- Reports should identify key risk factors and offer plausible theory that is situation based.
- The use of structured risk assessment guides can improve practice.
- Risk assessment should be linked directly to risk management practices. Therefore it is important that risk assessment and management is transferred into practice, as well as being seen as the cornerstone of practice.

All these authors' recommendations could clearly help to improve the mental health nurses' approach to the assessment and management of risk to others in their everyday practice.

The risk of assessing risk to others

This chapter cannot be complete without at least raising the issue of the effect on the patient of having an assessment of risk to others. Previously the author termed this '*the risk of risk assessment*' (Woods, in press):

> '*The results of risk assessment and related management plans can have a profound effect on those subject to these, resulting in labelling and stigmatisation. Hepworth (1982) clearly explained that there is a risk of the dangerous individual becoming a 'non-person' in therapeutic terms; and his/her dangerousness becomes based solely on previous recorded violence. Such an individual may well become static on the continuum of 'dangerous/non-dangerous' or 'person/non-person'. The other examples that clearly come to mind are where individuals have been labelled as a psychopath, having a personality disorder or the new term Dangerous and Severe Personality Disorder following assessment and consequences this can have when trying to access services at a later date and the stigma they will receive. One does not have to look hard in the literature to find many examples of this. The important message for mental health nurses to bear in mind in relation to this risk of risk assessment is that if your patient does not want to comply with your risk assessment is this the reason why.*'

Conclusion

This chapter has probably missed out more than it has covered as the assessment and management of risk to others is a complex and extensive subject area. Those reading this book need to consider how the principles suggested apply to their own practice area. Assessing risk to others cannot be considered an exact science. Researchers have tried for many years to uncover the complex relationships that exist between risk to others and demographic, clinical and contextual variables. Will they ever have clear answers for clinicians to use? It is sad to say but probably not. However, what they have done, and will continue to do, is determine some variables that consistently remain more associated in some patients than others.

Every mental health nurse can probably reflect and remember the patient that was admitted and before very long was violent or aggressive and one or a number of their colleagues were assaulted. Questions are always asked around 'Should we have known?' 'What if we had done this or done something another way?' or 'Are we to blame in some way? Whilst some of these questions are useful to reflect upon to develop practice, it is perhaps not constructive to lay any blame. Just one example that comes to mind is that nurses can sometimes fail to recognise the effects that substances can have up to a month after the person has taken them – a delayed reaction, as well as withdrawals – and many nurses do not pay enough attention to this aspect of substance misuse.

The assessment of risk to others needs to be a systematic process, where some patients are screened and others comprehensively assessed. Any risks identified need to be appropriately managed for all concerned. It is also vital that assessment of risk to others is not a one-off process or that mental health nurses do not become complacent with well-known patients; otherwise errors will undoubtedly occur more than they should by chance. The whole process of risk assessment and management in relation to risk to others was perhaps summed up over two decades ago by Scott (1977, p.129):

'Before factors can be considered they must be gathered. It is patience, thoroughness and persistence in this process, rather than any diagnostic or interviewing brilliance, that produces results. In this sense the telephone, the written requests for past records and the checking of information against other informants, are the important diagnostic devices.'

On a very final note, risk assessment and management cannot be separated by each other. Doyle and Dolan (2002, p.653) rightly state that *'evidence-based practice requires that the assessment of risk informs the management plan in a systematic fashion'.*

Acknowledgements

The author would like to kindly thank Wiley-Blackwell for permission to reproduce some of the text contained within this chapter that originally appeared in Woods and Ashley (2007) and Woods and Lasiuk (2008).

References

Aiken, G.J.M. (1984) Assaults on staff in a locked ward: prediction and consequences. *Medicine, Science, and the Law*, **24**(3), 199–207.

Anderson, T.R., Bell, C.C., Powell, T.E., Williamson, J.L. & Blount, M.A. Jr (2004) Assessing psychiatric patients for violence. *Community Mental Health Journal*, **40**(4), 379–399.

Appelbaum, P.S., Robbins, P.C. & Monahan, J. (2000) Violence and delusions: data from the MacArthur Risk Assessment Study. *American Journal of Psychiatry*, **157**, 566–572.

Appleby, L., Shaw, J., Kapur, N., *et al.* (2006) *Avoidable Deaths: Five Year Report by the National Confidential Inquiry into Suicide and Homicide by People with Mental Illness.* University of Manchester, Manchester. Available at http://www.medicine.manchester.ac.uk/suicideprevention/nci/Useful/avoidable_deaths_full_report.pdf (accessed 13 April 2008).

Aquilina, C. (1991) Violence by psychiatric inpatients. *Medicine, Science, and the Law*, **31**(4), 306–312.

Bensley, L., Nelson, N., Kaufman, J., Silverstein, B. Kalat, J., & Shields, J.W. (1997) Injuries due to assaults on psychiatric hospital employees in Washington State. *American Journal of Industrial Medicine*, **31**(1), 92–99.

Blomhoff, S., Siem, S. & Friis, S. (1990) Can prediction of violence among psychiatric inpatients be improved? *Hospital and Community Psychiatry*, **41**(7), 771–775.

Bloom, H., Webster, C., Hucker, S. & De Freitas, K. (2005) The Canadian contribution to violence risk assessment: history and implications for current psychiatric practice. *Canadian Journal of Psychiatry*, **50**(1), 3–11.

Blumenthal, S. & Lavender, T. (2001) *Violence and Mental Disorder: A Critical Aid to the Assessment and Management of Risk.* Jessica Kingsley, London.

Boer, D.P., Hart S.D., Kropp, P.R. & Webster, C.D. (1997) *Manual for the Sexual Violence Risk-20.* The British Columbia Institute Against Family Violence, co-published with the Mental Health, Law, and Policy Institute at Simon Fraser University, Burnaby, British Columbia.

Borum, R. (1996) Improving the clinical practice of violence risk assessment. *American Psychologist*, **51**(9), 945–956.

Borum, R., Otto, R., & Golding, S. (1993) Improving clinical judgment and decision making in forensic evaluation. *Journal of Psychiatry and Law*, **21**(1), 35–76.

Buchanan, A. (1997) The investigation of acting on delusions as a tool for risk assessment in the mentally disordered. *British Journal of Psychiatry*, **170** (Supplement 32), 12–16.

Collins, M. & Davies, S. (2005) The Security Needs Assessment Profile: a multidimensional approach to measuring security needs. *International Journal of Forensic Mental Health*, **4**(1), 39–52.

Cooper, A.F. & Mendonca, J.D. (1991) A prospective study of patient assaults on nurses in a provincial psychiatric hospital in Canada. *Acta Psychiatrica Scandinavica*, **84**(2), 163–166.

Cuffel, B.J., Shumway, M., Chouljian, T.L. & MacDonald, T. (1994) A longitudinal study of substance use and community violence in schizophrenia. *Journal of Nervous and Mental Disease*, **182**(12), 704–708.

Daffern, M. & Howells, K. (2002) Psychiatric inpatient aggression: a review of structural and functional assessment approaches. *Aggression and Violent Behavior*, **7**, 477–497.

Davies, S. (2001) Assaults and threats on psychiatrists. *Psychiatric Bulletin*, **25**, 89–91.

Dempster, R.J. & Hart, S.D. (2002) The relative utility of fixed and variable risk factors in discriminating sexual recidivists and nonrecidivists. *Sexual Abuse: Journal of Research and Treatment*, **14**(2), 121–138.

Department of Health (2007) *Best Practice in Managing Risk. Principles and Evidence for Best Practice in the Assessment and Management of Risk to Self and Others in Mental Health Services*. Department of Health, London.

Dittmann, V. (1996) Substance abuse, mental disorders and crime: comorbidity and multi-axial assessment in forensic psychiatry. *European Addiction Research*, **2**(1), 3–10.

Dolan, M., & Doyle, M. (2000) Violence risk prediction: clinical and actuarial measures and the role of the Psychopathy Checklist. *British Journal of Psychiatry*, **177**, 303–311.

Doyle, M. (1999) Organizational responses to crisis and risk: issues and implications for mental health nurses. In: *Managing Crisis and Risk in Mental Health Nursing* (ed. T. Ryan), pp. 40–56. Stanley Thornes, Cheltenham.

Doyle, M. & Dolan, M. (2002) Violence risk assessment: combining actuarial and clinical information to structure clinical judgments for the formulation and management of risk. *Journal of Psychiatric and Mental Health Nursing*, **9**(6), 649–657.

Doyle, M. & Duffy, D. (2006) Assessing and managing risk to self and others. In: *Forensic Mental Health Nursing: Interventions with People with 'Personality Disorder'* (National Forensic Nurses' Research and Development Group; eds P. Woods, A. Kettles, R. Byrt, *et al.*), pp. 135–150. Quay Books, London.

Drinkwater, J. & Gudjonsson, G.H. (1989) The nature of violence in psychiatric hospital. In: *Clinical Approaches to Violence* (eds K. Howells & C.R. Hollin), pp. 287–307. Wiley, New York.

D'Silva, K. & Ferriter, M. (2003) Substance use by the mentally disordered committing serious offences – a high-security hospital study. *Journal of Forensic Psychiatry and Psychology*, **14**(1), 178–193.

Edwards, J.G., Jones, D., Reid, W.H. & Chu, C.C. (1988) Physical assaults in a psychiatric unit of a general hospital. *American Journal of Psychiatry*, **145**, 1568–1571.

Fisher, W.A. (1994) Restraint and seclusion: a review of the literature. *American Journal of Psychiatry*, **151**, 1584–1591.

Flannery, R.B. Jr, Hanson, M.A. & Penk, W.E. (1994) Risk factors for psychiatric inpatient assaults on staff. *Journal of Mental Health Administration*, **21**(1), 24–31.

Fottrell, E. (1980) A study of violent behaviour among patients in psychiatric hospitals. *British Journal of Psychiatry*, **136**, 216–221.

Fottrell, E., Bewley, T. & Squizzonni, M.A. (1978) A study of aggressive and violent behavior among a group of inpatients. *Medicine, Science, and the Law*, **18**, 66–69.

Fulwiler, C., Grossman, H., Forbes, C. & Ruthazer, R. (1997) Early-onset substance abuse and community violence by outpatients with chronic mental illness. *Psychiatric Services*, **48**(9), 1181–1185.

Grove, W.M., Zald, D.H., Lebow, B.S., Snitz, B.E., & Nelson, C. (2000) Clinical versus mechanical prediction: a meta-analysis. *Psychological Assessment*, **12**(1), 19–30.

Häfner, H. & Böker, W. (1982) *Crimes of Violence of Mentally Abnormal Offenders*. Cambridge University Press, Cambridge.

Haller, R.M. & Deluty, R.H. (1988) Assaults on staff by psychiatric inpatients: a critical review. *British Journal of Psychiatry*, **152**, 174–179.

Harris, G. & Rice, M. (1997) Risk appraisal and management of violent behaviour. *Psychiatric Services*, **48**(9), 1168–1176.

Hart, S.D. (1998) The role of psychopathy in assessing risk for violence: conceptual and methodological issues. *Legal and Criminological Psychology*, **3**(1), 121–137.

Hellerstein, D., Frosch, W., & Koenigsberg, H.W. (1987) The clinical significance of command hallucinations. *American Journal of Psychiatry*, **144**, 219–221.

Hepworth, D. (1982) Influence of the concept of 'danger' on assessment of danger to self and others. *Medicine Science and the Law*, **22**(4), 245–254.

Hoptman, M.J., Yates, K.F., Patalinjug, M.B., Wack, R.C. & Convit, A. (1999) Clinical prediction of assaultive behavior among male psychiatric patients at a maximum-security forensic facility. *Psychiatric Services*, **50**, 1461–1466.

James, D.V., Fineberg, N.A., Shah, A.K. & Priest, R.G. (1990) An increase in violence on an acute psychiatric ward: a study of associated factors. *British Journal of Psychiatry*, **156**, 846–852.

Johnson, B.R. (2000) Assessing the risk factors for aggression. In: *New Directions for Mental Health Services, Psychiatric Aspects of Violence: Issues in Prevention and Treatment, No. 86* (ed. C.C. Bell). Jossey-Bass, San Francisco.

Johnson, M.E. (2004) Violence on inpatient psychiatric units: state of the science. *Journal of the American Psychiatric Nurses Association*, **10**(3), 113–121.

Junginger, J. (1995) Command hallucinations and the prediction of dangerousness. *Psychiatric Services*, **46**, 911–914.

Junginger, J., Parks-levy, J. & McGuire, L. (1998) Delusions and symptom-consistent violence. *Psychiatric Services*, **49**, 218–220.

Kaspar, M.E., Rogers, R., & Adams, P.A. (1996) Dangerousness and command hallucinations: an investigation of psychiatric inpatients. *Bulletin of the American Academy of Psychiatry and Law*, **24**, 219–224.

Kettles, A.M. (2004) A concept analysis of forensic risk. *Journal of Psychiatric and Mental Health Nursing*, **11**(4), 484–493.

Krakowski, M., Convit, A., Jaeger, J., Shang, L. & Volavka, J. (1989) Neurological impairment in violent schizophrenic inpatients. *American Journal of Psychiatry*, **146**(7), 849–853.

Larkin, E., Murtagh, S. & Jones, S. (1988) A preliminary study of violent incidents in a special hospital (Rampton). *British Journal of Psychiatry*, **153**, 226–231.

Lewis, A.H.O. & Webster, C.D. (2004) General instruments for risk assessment. *Current Opinion in Psychiatry*, **17**(5), 401–405.

Lidz, C.W., Mulvey, E.P. & Gardner, W. (1993) The accuracy of predictions of violence to others. *Journal of the American Medical Association*, **269**, 1007–1011.

Link, B.G. & Stueve, A. (1994) Psychotic symptoms and the violent/illegal behaviour of mental patients compared to community controls. In: *Violence and Mental Disorder: Developments in Risk Assessment* (eds J. Monahan & H.J. Steadman). Chicago University Press, Chicago.

Link, B.G., Stueve, A. & Phelan, A. (1998) Psychotic symptoms and violent behaviors: probing the components of 'threat/control-override' symptoms. *Social Psychiatry and Psychiatric Epidemiology*, **33**, S55–S60.

Maclean, Lord (2000) *Report of the Committee on Serious and Violent Sexual Offenders*. Scottish Executive, Edinburgh.

Mawson, D. (1990) Violence in hospital. In: *Principles and Practice of Forensic Psychiatry* (eds R. Bluglass & P. Bowden), pp. 641–648. Churchill Livingstone, Edinburgh.

McNiel, D. & Binder, R. (1994) Screening for risk of inpatient violence: validation of an actuarial tool. *Law and Human Behavior*, **18**(5), 579–586.

McNiel, D.E., Binder, R.L. & Greenfield, T.K. (1988) Predictors of violence in civilly committed acute psychiatric patients. *American Journal of Psychiatry*, **145**, 965–970.

Miller, R.J., Zadolinnyj, K. & Hafner, R.F. (1993) Profiles and predictors of assaultiveness for different psychiatric ward populations. *American Journal of Psychiatry*, **150**, 1368–1373.

Monahan, J. (1981) *The Clinical Prediction of Violent Behavior*. National Institute of Mental Health, Rockville.

Monahan, J. (1984) The prediction of violent behavior: toward a second generation of theory and policy. *American Journal of Psychiatry*, **141**, 10–15.

Monahan, J. (1988) Risk assessment of violence among the mentally disordered: generating useful knowledge. *International Journal of Law and Psychiatry*, **11**(3), 249–257.

Monahan, J. (1993) Limiting therapist exposure to Tarasoff liability: guidelines for risk containment. *American Psychologist*, **48**, 242–250.

Monahan, J. & Steadman, H.J. (1994) Towards a rejuvenation of risk assessment research. In: *Violence and Mental Disorder: Developments in Risk Assessment* (eds J. Monahan & H.J. Steadman), pp. 1–17. University of Chicago Press, Chicago.

Monahan, J., Steadman, H.J., Silver, E., *et al.* (2001) *Rethinking Risk Assessment: The MacArthur Study of Mental Disorder and Violence*. Oxford University Press, Oxford.

Morgan, S. (2000) *Clinical Risk Management: A Tool and Practitioner Manual*. Sainsbury Centre for Mental Health, London.

Morgan, S. & Hemming, M. (1999) Balancing care and control: risk management and compulsory community treatment. *Mental Health and Learning Disabilities Care*, **3**(1), 19–21.

Morgan, S. & Wetherell, A. (2004) Assessing and managing risk. In: *The Art and Science of Mental Health Nursing: A Textbook of Principles and Practice* (eds I. Norman & I. Ryrie), pp. 208–240. Open University Press, Maidenhead.

Morrison, E.F. (1998) The culture of caregiving and aggression in psychiatric settings. *Archives of Psychiatric Nursing*, **12**, 21–31.

Mossman, D. (1994) Assessing predictions of violence: being accurate about accuracy. *Journal of Consulting and Clinical Psychology*, **62**(4), 783–792.

Mullen, P.E. (1997) A reassessment of the link between mental disorder and violent behaviour, and its implications for clinical practice. *Australian and New Zealand Journal of Psychiatry*, **31**, 3–11.

National Institute for Health and Clinical Excellence (2005) *Violence: The Short-term Management of Disturbed/Violent Behaviour in In-Patient Psychiatric Settings and Emergency Departments*. Clinical Guideline 25. NICE, London.

Needham, I., Abderhalden, C., Meer, R., Dassen, T., Haug, H.J., Halfens, R.J.G. & Fischer, J.E. (2004) The effectiveness of two interventions in the management of patient violence in acute mental inpatient settings: report on a pilot study. *Journal of Psychiatric and Mental Health Nursing*, **11**(5), 595–601.

Noble, P. & Rodger, S. (1989) Violence by psychiatric inpatients. *British Journal of Psychiatry*, **155**, 384–390.

Norko, M.A. & Baranoski, M.V. (2005) The state of contemporary risk assessment research. *Canadian Journal of Psychiatry*, **50**(1), 18–26.

Otto, R. (2000) Assessing and managing violence risk in outpatient settings. *Journal of Clinical Psychology*, **56**(10), 1239–1262.

Owen, C., Tarantello, C., Jones, M. & Tennant, C. (1998a) Violence and aggression in psychiatric units. *Psychiatric Services*, **49**, 1452–1457.

Owen, C., Tarantello, C., Jones, M. & Tennant, C. (1998b) Repetitively violent patients in psychiatric units. *Psychiatric Services*, **49**, 1458–1461.

Pearson, M., Wilmot, E. & Padi, M. (1986) A study of violent behaviour among in-patients in a psychiatric hospital. *British Journal of Psychiatry*, **149**, 232–235.

Phillips, P. (2000) Substance misuse, offending and mental illness: a review. *Journal of Psychiatric and Mental Health Nursing*, **7**(6), 483–489.

Pollock, N. & Webster, C. (1990) The clinical assessment of dangerousness. In: *Principles and Practice of Forensic Psychiatry* (eds R. Bluglass & P. Bowden), pp. 489–497. Churchill Livingstone, Edinburgh.

Rabinowitz, J. & Garelik-Wyler, R. (1999) Accuracy and confidence in clinical assessment of psychiatric inpatients' risk of violence. *International Journal of Law and Psychiatry*, **22**(1), 99–106.

Reid, W.H., Bollinger, M.F. & Edwards, J.G. (1989) Serious assaults by inpatients. *Psychosomatics*, **30**, 54–56.

Rice, M.E., Harris, G.T. & Quinsey, V.L. (2002) The appraisal of violence risk. *Current Opinion in Psychiatry*, **15**(6), 589–593.

Rudnick, A. (1999) Relation between command hallucinations and dangerous behaviour. *Journal of the American Academy of Psychiatry and the Law*, **27**, 253–257.

Scott, P. (1977) Assessing dangerousness in criminals. *British Journal of Psychiatry*, **131**(2), 127–142.

Shah, A.K., Fineberg, N.A. & James, D.V. (1991) Violence among psychiatric inpatients. *Acta Psychiatrica Scandinavica*, **84**(4), 305–309.

Snowden, P. (1997) Practical aspects of clinical risk assessment and management. *British Journal of Psychiatry*, **170** (Supplement 32), 32–34.

Soliman, A.E.D. & Reza, H. (2001) Risk factors and correlates of violence among acutely ill adult psychiatric inpatients. *Psychiatric Services*, **52**, 75–80.

Soyka, M. (2000) Substance misuse, psychiatric disorder and violent and disturbed behaviour. *British Journal of Psychiatry*, **176**, 345–350.

Steadman, H.J. & Cocozza, J.J. (1974) *Careers of the Criminally Insane: Excessive Social Control of Deviance*. Lexington Books, Lexington.

Steadman, H.J., Silver, E., Monahan, J., *et al.* (2000) A classification tree approach to the development of actuarial violence risk assessment tools. *Law and Human Behavior*, **24**(1), 83–100.

Steinert, T. (2001) Mental disorder, criminality and violence: knowledge and consequences. *Recht & Psychiatrie*, **19**(2), 89–96.

Steinert, T., Wölfle, M. & Gebhardt, R.-P. (2000) Measurement of violence during in-patient treatment and association with psychopathology. *Acta Psychiatrica Scandinavica*, **102**, 107–112.

Stompe, T., Ortwein-Swoboda, Q. & Schand, H. (2004) Schizophrenia, delusional symptoms, and violence: the threat/control-override concept reexamined. *Schizophrenia Bulletin*, **30**(1), 31–44.

Swanson, J.W., Holzer, C.E., Ganju, V.K. & Jono, R.T. (1990) Violence and psychiatric disorder in the community: evidence from the Epidemiologic Catchment Area Studies. *Hospital and Community Psychiatry*, **41**, 761–770.

Swanson, J.W., Borum, R., Swartz, M.S. & Monahan, J. (1996) Psychotic symptoms and disorders and the risk of violent behaviour in the community. *Criminal Behaviour and Mental Health*, **6**, 309–329.

Swanson, J., Estroff, S., Swartz, M., Borum, R., Lachicotte, W., Zimmer, C. & Wagner, R. (1997) Violence and severe mental disorder in clinical and community populations: the effects of psychotic symptoms, comorbidity and lack of treatment. *Psychiatry*, **60**, 1–22.

Tardiff, K. (1984) Characteristics of assaultive patients in private hospitals. *American Journal of Psychiatry*, **141**, 1232–1235.

Tardiff, K. & Sweillam, A. (1982) Assaultive behavior among chronic inpatients. *American Journal of Psychiatry*, **139**(2), 212–215.

Taylor, P.J. (1985) Motives for offending among violent and psychotic men. *British Journal of Psychiatry*, **147**, 491–498.

Taylor, P.J., Garety, P., Buchanan, A., Reed, A., Wessely, S. & Ray, K. (1994) Delusions and violence. In: *Violence and Mental Disorder: Developments in Risk Assessment* (eds J. Monahan & H.J. Steadman), pp. 161–182. University of Chicago Press, Chicago.

Taylor, P.J., Leese, M., Williams, D., Butwell, M., Daly, R. & Larkin, E. (1998) Mental disorder and violence. A special (high security) hospital study. *British Journal of Psychiatry*, **172**, 218–226.

The Audit Team, Royal College of Psychiatrists' Centre for Quality Improvement (2007a) *Healthcare Commission National Audit of Violence 2006–7: Final Report – Working Age Adult Services*. Royal College of Psychiatrists, London. Available at http://www.rcpsych.ac.uk/researchandtrainingunit/centreforqualityimprovement/nationalauditofviolence/navnationalreports.aspx (accessed 7 April 2008).

The Audit Team, Royal College of Psychiatrists' Centre for Quality Improvement (2007b) *Healthcare Commission National Audit of Violence 2006–7: Final Report – Older People's Services*. Royal College of Psychiatrists, London. Available at http://www.rcpsych.ac.uk/researchandtrainingunit/

centreforqualityimprovement/nationalauditofviolence/navnationalreports.
aspx (accessed 7 April 2008).

Wallace, C., Mullen, P.E. & Burgess, P. (2004) Criminal offending in schizophrenia over a 25-year period marked by deinstitutionalization and
increasing prevalence of comorbid substance use disorders. *American
Journal of Psychiatry*, **161**(4), 716–727.

Webster, C.D., Douglas, K.S., Eaves, D. & Hart, S.D. (1997) Assessing risk of
violence to others. In: *Impulsivity: Theory, Assessment, and Treatment* (eds
C.D. Webster & M.A. Jackson), pp. 251–277. Guilford Press, New York.

Wellman, N. (2006) Assessing risk. In: *Working with Serious Mental Illness:
A Manual for Clinical Practice* (eds C. Gamble & G. Brennan), 2nd edn,
pp. 145–164. Elsevier, Edinburgh.

Wetherell, A. (2001) Risk in mental health – part 3. *Breakthrough*, **7**(1), 15–16.

Woods, P. (2001) Risk assessment and management. In: *Forensic Mental Health:
Issues in Practice* (eds C. Dale, T. Thompson & P. Woods), pp. 85–97.
Bailliere Tindall, Edinburgh.

Woods, P. (in press) The forensic mental health nurse's role in risk assessment, measurement and management. In: *Forensic Nursing: Roles,
Capabilities and Competencies* (National Forensic Nurses' Research and
Development Group; eds A. Kettles, P. Woods & R. Byrt, *et al.*), Chapter 10. Quay Books, London.

Woods, P. & Ashley, C. (2007) Violence and aggression: a literature review.
Journal of Psychiatric and Mental Health Nursing, **14**(7), 652–660.

Woods, P. & Lasiuk, G. (2008) Risk prediction: a review of the literature.
Journal of Forensic Nursing, **4**(1), 1–11.

Wright, S., Gray, R., Parkes, J. & Gournay, K. (2002a) *The Recognition,
Prevention and Therapeutic Management of Violence in Acute In-Patient
Psychiatry: A Literature Review and Evidence-Based Recommendations for Good
Practice*. United Kingdom Central Council for Nursing, Midwifery and
Health Visiting, London.

Wright, S., Gournay, K., Glorney, E. & Thornicroft, G. (2002b) Mental
illness, substance abuse, demographics and offending: dual diagnosis
in the suburbs. *Journal of Forensic Psychiatry*, **13**(1), 35–52.

Chapter 6

Risk to Self

B. Lee Murray and Eve Upshall

Introduction

Risk to self includes:

- suicidal behaviour (varying degrees of self-harm, including self-injurious behaviour and self-mutilation);
- self-neglect (both physical and social);
- vulnerability (being at risk of harm from others).

The related issues will be examined in the context of gender, culture, development and the nurse–patient relationship. This chapter reflects on the biological, psychological and social theories of risk to self and discusses this risk in the context of the determinants of health. This chapter also contains information nurses can use to understand risk to self behaviours and tools to provide appropriate care related to assessment, nursing diagnosis, care planning, intervention and evaluation.

Suicidal behaviour

The most obvious and catastrophic aspect of risk to self is suicide and self-harm behaviour. Suicidal behaviour is complex and involves many aspects of an individual's personality, state of health and life circumstances (Tondo and Baldessarini 2001). Many lives are touched by a completed suicide and many people struggle with what to do when a person is identified as suicidal. Self-harm and suicidal behaviour can be one of the most challenging behaviours for nurses and other healthcare professionals to address. A widely held view is that being suicidal is itself a psychopathological condition or an indicator of mental illness. In fact psychological autopsies have found evidence of psychopathology in as many as 90% of completed suicides (Conwell and Henderson 1996).

Certainly someone considering a form of suicidal behaviour is in a depressed mood, but this state of mind does not necessarily represent a psychiatric diagnosis, as it may be a reaction to psychosocial issues and adverse life circumstances. Usually a distinction can be made between suicide as a consequence of a pre-existing mental illness and suicide as a response to a difficult or intolerable life situation in the absence of a psychiatric diagnosis (Tondo 2000). In fact 30.1% of all persons with suicidal ideation do not have a defined mental disorder, and 21.5% do not even have a sub-threshold disorder (Ahrens *et al.* 2000). This leaves us with the question: *Is it possible to distinguish between suicide as a symptom, a disorder or an outcome of illness?* Experts in the field suggest that someone considering suicide is in so much pain that they feel they have no other option (NANYouth 2004). The state of mind of someone considering suicidal behaviour has been described as hopeless, helpless, powerless and filled with self-hatred and rejection. As a way to release this pain and the burden they perceive as having placed on others, they, in desperation, opt for death (NANYouth 2004).

Other literature indicates that suicide ideation and behaviour should be regarded as a symptom and is often a means of communicating that life has become difficult and intolerable (Levenkron 1998; Ahrens *et al.* 2000; Machoian 2001; Murray 2003). Therefore it is important for nurses to listen to these attempts to communicate and to begin to understand the meaning of the self-harm and suicidal behaviour. Despite recent efforts to identify risk factors and protective factors for suicidal behaviour, our ability to make an accurate prediction of suicide is limited. An early comprehensive assessment of risk is crucial in understanding the meaning of the behaviour, and guiding interventions to prevent escalation or chronicity of the behaviour (Murray 2003). A thorough assessment guides the intervention and must be implemented in the context of the patient's family, social world and broader community. Establishment of a trusting relationship between the nurse and the suicidal patient is imperative for accurate assessment and effective interventions.

Suicide is highly preventable and yet it persists. Tondo and Baldessarini (2001) also point out that the knowledge on which to base sound clinical and public policy regarding suicide prevention and treatment still remains limited. Self-harm and suicidal behaviour continues and suicides are still being carried out to completion. Because those at risk of suicide appear in most healthcare settings, nurses are in a unique position to prevent death by suicide. Nurses must be able to engage and connect with the suicidal patient and complete a comprehensive assessment of risk to guide appropriate interventions. They must also know what to do when working with a patient who is acutely suicidal.

There are a number of concepts that are generally understood in relation to risk to self. Definitions of these are provided in Box 6.1.

Box 6.1 Key definitions in relation to risk to self.

- **Self-harm** is '*the various methods by which individuals injure themselves, such as self-laceration, self-battering, taking overdoses or exhibiting deliberate recklessness*' (United States Department of Health and Human Services 2001, p.202).

- **Suicide** is the voluntary act of killing oneself. It is sometimes called *suicide completion*. The behavioural definition of suicide is limited and does not consider the complexity of the underlying depressive illness, personal motivations, and situational and family factors that provoke the suicide act.

- **Parasuicide** is a voluntary attempt to kill oneself. It is frequently called *attempted suicide*. Parasuicidal behaviour varies by intent (Ferreira de Castro *et al.* 1998). For example, some people who attempt suicide truly wish to die, but others simply wish to feel nothing for a while. Still others attempt suicide because they want to send a message to others that life is difficult due to their psychosocial issues and their resulting emotional state.

- **Suicidal ideation** is thinking about harming one's self and/or planning one's own death. Suicidal behaviour can be identified along a continuum of low to high risk. Suicidal ideation poses the lowest risk, with very lethal means at a planned time of aloneness posing the highest risk. A risk/rescue ratio also must be taken into consideration. The likelihood of rescue becomes part of the calculation of risk. The more lethal the means, the less likely the person will be rescued.

- **Lethality** '*refers to the probability that a person will complete suicide. Lethality is determined by the seriousness of the person's intent and the likelihood that the planned method will result in death. High lethality includes firearms, hanging, carbon monoxide poisoning, drowning, suffocation or jumping from a great height*' (Murray and Hauenstein 2008, p.901).

- **Risk/rescue ratio** '*refers to the lethality of means and the likelihood of rescue. Suicidal risk carries with it a progression of seriousness from suicidal ideation to completed suicide. Risk is lowest when intent is weak and the method used has low lethality. The likelihood of rescue is dependent upon communication of intent and lower lethality of means*' (Murray and Hauenstein 2008, p.901).

- **Hopelessness** '*is a perception of having no hope that one's life situation/circumstance will change or improve. It is characterized by feelings of inadequacy and an inability to act on one's own behalf*' (Murray and Hauenstein 2008, p.900).

- **Helplessness** '*is the perception of having limited ability or ambition to change one's current life situation. A sense of being unable to help oneself and a sense that there is a lack of support or protection*' (Murray and Hauenstein 2008, p.900).

- **Powerlessness** '*is the perception of having no power or control over one's life circumstance. A belief that the world will never be fair. Lacking strength or power; helpless and totally ineffectual. Lacking legal or other authority*' (Murray and Hauenstein 2008, p.900).

Terminology

The terms self-harm, self-mutilation and self-injurious behaviour have been used interchangeably in the literature. The various labels have made it confusing for mental health professionals to understand behaviours that have also been defined as suicidal (Murray 2003). Deliberate self-harm has been defined as any suicide attempt (Aoun 1999). Deliberate self-harm according to Rioch (1995) includes behaviours where the individual can be considered suicidal (or engaging in suicidal behaviour) such as taking an overdose, self-suffocation, self-strangulation, wrist cutting and drowning. However, Anderson (1999) indicated that the term 'attempted suicide' is weak because it does not consider that some people do not have the intention of killing themselves. Anderson indicates that the term deliberate self-harm is also used to refer to behaviours that may be fatal but where suicide may not have been the intention. In comparison, gestured suicide includes behaviour that resembles suicide but in which the person did not intend to die (Fairbairn 1995). Self-harm is often both impulsive and compulsive (Favaro and Santonastaso 2000). Self-mutilation is a form of self-injurious and self-harm behaviour and is described as:

'. . . the act of damaging seriously by cutting, cutting off, or altering an essential part of the body usually the skin' (Levenkron 1998, p.22).

Research indicates that self-harm behaviour is often a means of communication (Halliday and Mackrell 1998; Machoian 2001). This is particularly true for adolescents who are struggling with particular problems, stressors and life events and who exhibit self-harm behaviour as a means of communication or a way of coping (Murray and Wright 2006). Some adolescents indicate that they cut as a way to release tension and achieve calmness; others indicate it is a means of punishing themselves or others; still others indicate it is a way of putting the internal psychological pain on the outside so they can see and feel it in a physiological sense. However, most adolescents indicate that self-mutilation is a way of telling others that something is very wrong in their lives. It is also a way of letting others know that their life has become unbearable and they assume no one understands the seriousness of their problems.

Self-harm behaviour may sometimes be interpreted by professionals as attention-seeking behaviour and is often looked upon unfavourably, and thus there is a tendency to ignore the behaviour. If we assume the behaviour is a way of communication and we ignore the behaviour we only escalate the behaviour. Intervention needs to focus on assisting patients to use more appropriate means to receive the attention they need and the attention they deserve. A caring and engaging approach that includes active listening often de-escalates the behaviour.

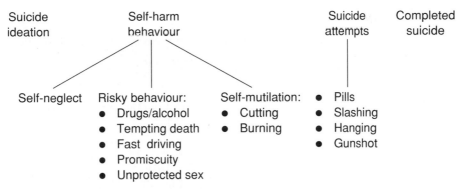

Vulnerability is risk to self, related to potential harm from others.

Figure 6.1   Risk to self as a continuum.

At-risk behaviour is also a form of self-harm. Fast and reckless driving, putting oneself in danger, promiscuity, unprotected sex and drug and alcohol abuse are a few examples of at-risk behaviour. This often indicates that life is not worth living and the individual does not feel worthy of self-care, and has no regard for personal safety or self-preservation.

Risk to self may be viewed on a continuum (see Figure 6.1). The chapter is developed in the context of this conceptual view.

Epidemiology

Barring the very young, suicide occurs in all cultures, age groups and social classes. In 2000, the worldwide prevalence of completed suicide was 815,000, a rate of 1 death every 40 seconds or 14.5 deaths per 100,000 (WHO 2002). It is suspected that rates are higher than reported as they can be disguised as motor vehicle accidents and homicides (Kohlmeier *et al.* 2001). In general, rates are higher for men and for those over the age of 60. On average, there are about three completed suicides by men for every suicide completion by women and three times the number of people over the age of 60 completed suicide compared to those aged 15–29 (WHO 2002). The rates of men may be higher as they tend to use more lethal means such as firearms (Tondo and Baldessarini 2001). However, the rate of attempted suicide worldwide is 10–20 times higher than completion, resulting in 1 attempt every 3 seconds (WHO 2002), with women more likely to attempt and not complete.

In Canada, the rate of suicide in 2004 was 11.3 per 100,000 (Statistics Canada 2008), greater than accidents and homicides combined (Cutliffe 2003), with rates in the mid to high range as compared worldwide (WHO 2002). The most common means of death were by hanging, poisoning and firearms (Statistics Canada 2006). In 2004 there were 32,439 deaths attributed to suicide in the US; a rate of 11.0 per 100,000 (Minino *et al.* 2007) which registers suicide as the 11th leading cause of death. The most common means of suicide were by firearm, suffocation and poisoning. In 2004 the numbers of suicides accounted for 1% of all deaths in the UK. This was reflected in a rate of 18.1 per 100,000 for men and 6.0 per 100,000 for women who completed suicide in the UK, reiterating that suicide is still a major public health concern especially in young men (Brock *et al.* 2006). Scotland had suicide rates that were consistently higher than the rates for other parts of the UK from 2002–2004 (Brock *et al.* 2006). The suicide rate for men in Wales was also higher than the overall UK rate across this period, as was that for Northern Ireland.

McAllister (2003) indicates that statistics on the prevalence and incidence of self-harm are unreliable due to the social taboo surrounding it. Many occurrences will not become known to professionals and will be treated in some other way. Indeed many people will deliberately avoid referral to mental health services even when they have been treated in emergency departments. Furthermore, she states that some professionals when aware of self-harm may even refuse to label this for fear of stigmatisation of their client.

Self-harm is a major public health problem in the UK, it is the most common reason for admission to hospital, it accounts for around 170,000 hospital attendances each year, and the incidence is increasing (Kapur *et al.* 1998; Kapur 2005). Many of those that self-harm repeat this behaviour within the next 12 months (Hawton *et al.* 1997; Owens *et al.* 2002; Zahl and Hawton 2004). Self-harm has been found to be more common in females (for example, Hawton 2000; O'Loughlin and Sherwood 2005).

Suicide is highly preventable and yet approximately 56% of people complete suicide on their first attempt (Isometsa and Lonnqvist 1998), and 25% of people hospitalised for attempted suicide kill themselves 3 months following discharge (Appleby *et al.* 1999a). People attempt suicide because others do not recognise the signs, an underlying major depressive disorder is not treated, or those with suicidal ideation fear the social stigma of discussing their problems. Cutliffe (2003) suggests the custodial practices, such as restricting freedom, continuous observation and removing dangerous objects, seen in psychiatric healthcare agencies are similar to policing practices which do little to address the root of the problem or alter suicidal ideation. Furthermore, because those at risk of suicidal behaviour appear in most healthcare settings, nurses are in a unique position to prevent death by suicide. Nurses must be able to assist a patient's potential for risk to self, determine its causes and identify factors that enhance its risk. They must know what to do when working with a patient who is acutely suicidal. The nurse can help to demystify suicide and destigmatise those at risk through individual and public education.

Etiology

'The convergence of physiologic, psychological and social factors can be directly linked to suicidal behaviour' (Murray and Hauenstein 2008, p.905). The idea that a person's social environment greatly influences suicidal and self-harm behaviour is consistently threaded throughout the literature (Adam *et al.* 1994). How these societal influences initiate the chain of events that lead to suicide and self-harm is controversial. Therefore, prevention must address the many psychological, biological and social stressors that are unmanageable and exceed typical coping effort, if it is to be effective (United States Department of Health and Human Services 2001). Those who are vulnerable typically lack the effective coping abilities which add to their vulnerability and increase their engagement in risky behaviours, often used in an effort to cope with stress. Risky behaviours for suicide include fast cars, tempting death, promiscuity, use of alcohol or drugs and purchase of a handgun.

Most who attempt suicide have seen a healthcare professional 1 month prior to the attempt (Blumenthal and Kupfer 1990), providing nurses with the opportunity and responsibility to assess, intervene and provide appropriate treatment to those who are at risk of suicidal ideation and behaviour. A comprehensive assessment identifies the physical, psychological and social factors that contribute to feelings of self-harm. These include changes in central nervous system (CNS) neurotransmitters, engaging in negative thinking and behaviours and deterioration of social relationships. Appropriate interventions guided by a comprehensive assessment of risk at this point can greatly reduce the likelihood of suicidal behaviour.

Biologic theories

Biological theories of suicide focus on the association between physical illness, the increased risk and the neurobiological component of suicide (Holkup 2003). The stress of physical illness can lead to depression and thoughts of whether life is worth living. It has been noted that many of the individuals who commit suicide have visited their healthcare provider with somatic complaints within months or days of completing suicide (Blumenthal and Kupfer 1990; Holkup 2003). *'Suicidal behaviour may also be a direct result of mood disorders such as major depressive disorder, which is exceedingly common in both Western and developing nations'* (Murray and Hauenstein 2008).

Psychiatric illness and sociological issues

Psychiatric illness is most often an ongoing risk factor, but the timing of suicidal acts tends to be associated with stressful life events, particularly those involving losses, separations and other changes or threats to self-esteem and confidence (Tondo and Baldessarini 2001). Major affective illnesses or mood disorders (major depressive and bipolar manic-depressive disorders) are associated with about half of all suicides (Tondo and Baldessarini 2001). Among those with major mood disorders, suicide accounted for 9–15% of deaths; however, those with milder illnesses that did not require hospitalisation had rates as low as 4% (Roy 1989; Clark and Goebel-Fabbri 1998; Bostwick and Pankratz 2000). However, state of mind does not necessarily represent psychiatric disorder and it is important to delineate between suicide as a consequence of pre-existing psychiatric illness and suicide as a response to a precipitating experience in the absence of a psychiatric disturbance (Tondo 2000).

Alcohol and substance use disorders are primary risk factors for suicide (Friedman 2006), are found in approximately 25% of suicides, and the life-time risk of suicide associated with substance abusers is similar to that associated with diagnosis of depression (Roy 1989; Clark and Goebel-Fabbri 1998). Furthermore, the risk of suicide is increased by a factor of six in personality disorders like borderline and antisocial personality disorder (Foster *et al.* 1999). Those with multiple co-morbid problems such as affective or psychotic disorders combined with drug or alcohol abuse are at the highest risk of suicide (Roy 1989; Mosciki 1998; Angst *et al.* 1999; Appleby *et al.* 1999b; Baldessarini *et al.* 1999). Anxiety disorders, even after controlling for co-morbid depression and substance abuse, account for 15–20% of suicides, while psychotic disorders such as schizophrenia account for a further 10–15% of suicides (Roy 1989).

Genetic abnormalities in the serotonergic neurotransmitter system may be responsible for the heightened familial risk of suicide (Mann *et al.* 2001). Serotonin is associated with poor impulse control and with the tendency to engage in violent and aggressive behaviour, and has been found to exist in deficient levels in individuals who have attempted suicide. Low levels of serotonin are also associated with depressive disorders, and thus this is one of the possible explanations of the strong link to suicide (Parris 2006). However, only about half of people who attempt suicide have clinical depression and there are other psychiatric illnesses that increase the risk of suicide (Meyer *et al.* 2003).

'Child abuse has been described as a specific vulnerability for psychopathology and suicide (MacMillan et al. 2001). Enhanced vulnerability to major depressive disorder and suicide associated with child abuse apparently are attributable to changes in the hypothalamic-pituitary-adrenal axis caused by intractable stress

and altered serotonin and dopamine metabolism (Skodol et al. 2002). Evidence from twin studies suggests that the link between childhood sexual abuse and biological alterations contributing to psychopathology may be independent of other environmental influences' (Murray and Hauenstein 2008, p.905).

Psychological theories

Suicidal individuals are found to have experienced a high level of stress for a prolonged period of time, with increasing levels in the time leading up to their suicidal action (Marriage and Family Encyclopedia 2008). Some psychologists believe suicidal behaviour occurs as an escape from this high-level stress and the resulting psychological pain (Parris 2006). It is hypothesised that this pain comes from prolonged frustration due to the inability of meeting or attaining basic psychological human needs such as the need for achievement, esteem, belonging, acceptance, love and safety (Parris 2006). Suicidal individuals are found to have few resources, and the resources that they have are often unavailable (Lester 2000). The lack of resources which leads to the inability to meet these needs leads to such negative emotional states as:

- shame, guilt, anger and grief (Marriage and Family Encyclopedia 2008);
- intense preoccupation with humiliation and disappointment (Leenaars 1998);
- intolerable aloneness and isolation (Adler and Buie 1996);
- punitive and aggressive impulses of revenge, spite or self-sacrifice;
- wishes to kill and be killed;
- yearning for release into a better experience through death (Tondo and Baldessarini 2001).

'Psychodynamic theories designate conflicts, losses and changes in relationships as contributors to suicidal risk and view suicide as a depressive or psychotic act, sometimes associated with fantasies of escape, reward, reunion and resurrection (Hendin 1991). Cognitive approaches also attribute suicide to learned impotence and hopelessness as an automatic and pervasive pathological scheme for organizing and interpreting experience (Beck et al. 1979a, Rosenberg 1993). The widely used cognitive theory of depression espoused by Aaron Beck and his associates (Beck et al. 1979b) accounts for how negative thoughts occur and how they can lead to suicidal behaviour' (Murray and Hauenstein 2008, p.906).

According to this theory, negative dysfunctional thoughts and beliefs lead to the cognitive changes noted earlier. Depressed people view themselves, their current situation and their future negatively. They are pessimistic about themselves as people and their ability to effect change, believe that others view them negatively and see no likelihood of improvement in their situation. People who engage in negative thinking believe that:

- 'No one is ever there for me';
- 'Nothing I do makes any difference';
- 'My future is very bleak'.

These thoughts tend to be spontaneous, repetitive, intrusive and ultimately powerful motivators of suicidal behaviour.

As Jamison (1999) noted, people who attempt or complete suicide often have difficult relationships with the people in their lives. Attachment theory can explain the social isolation and disrupted interpersonal relationships that are part of the spectrum of suicide (Lopez and Brennan 2000). In this theory, adult behaviour is explained by early interactions with the primary caregiver during infancy. Disrupted attachment results in the inability to form meaningful relationships with others or constant worry about the viability of a lasting relationship. Suicidal behaviour is viewed as the consequence of conflicted or distant relationships as an adult and the social isolation this often produces (Eng *et al.* 2002).

Tondo (2000) suggests a common theme: the ultimate defence of identity and the self. These themes can be found in several psychological interpretations of suicide from profound threats (losses and disappointments to self-esteem and confidence over persons, social groups or occupational activities in which much has been invested emotionally). These threats in turn lead to a sense of pervasive and irreparable damage to the self.

Social theories

Sociologically structured models of influences on suicide include family, culture, religion, occupation, socioeconomic class and groups or organisations (Tondo and Baldessarini 2001).

Socio-cultural etiology of risk to self

Tajfel and Turner (1979) and Hogg and Abrams (1988) defined social influence in terms of group norms, the ways in which the attitudes and behaviours of significant others (e.g. friends and peers) affect the decision to act in certain ways. This influence is distinct from social pressure from significant others to engage in a behaviour (i.e. injunctive norms). Terry *et al.* (2000) found that group identification moderated the group (descriptive) norms–behaviour relationship. The stronger a person identified with the groups, the more predictive the group behaviour was of individual behaviour. In turn, attitudes, subjective norms and perceived behavioural control are thought to determine behavioural intention. Attitudes are positive or negative evaluations of objects or behaviours. Subjective norms are measures of the perceived social pressure to engage or disengage in a behaviour (O'Connor *et al.* 2006). However, past behaviour is a consistent predictor of future behaviour (Sheeran *et al.* 1999; Armitage 2005; O'Connor *et al.* 2006). Moreover, social policies, such as access to gun control, have been shown to influence rates of suicide completion; since many suicides are acts of impulsivity, restrictions on access to such lethal weapons decrease the chances of fatality (Parris 2006).

Socioeconomic status

Suicidal behaviour is more common at either extreme of the socioeconomic continuum and the risk of suicide increases with a marked change, either up or down, in status. Level of education also plays a role in suicide risk; those with very high or very low levels are at lower risk (Tondo and Baldessarini 2001). Unemployment may also pose an indirect risk of suicide via family tension arising from loss of income and a normal social role. This loss may then lead to indignity, isolation, hopelessness, alcohol abuse and violence (Platt 1993). Social policy also can affect suicide rates; Zimmerman (2002) found a strong association between diminished state spending on welfare and suicide.

Religion

Religion may be a protective or risk factor related to risk to self.

> *'Rates of suicide vary considerably among religions and between regions that have a predominant religious culture; however, most religions are opposed to suicide'* (Murray and Hauenstein 2008, p.907).

Neeleman (1998) suggests that those who have higher rates of participation in religious practices may have lower risk of suicide. However, the guilt related to suicide in certain religions may contribute to increased risk to self. Similarly, religious groups with built-in social structures have been shown to play a role in the risk of attempting suicide. Populations affiliated with religions that offer great networks of emotional support, such as Catholicism, generally tend to have lower rates of suicide (Parris 2006).

Suicide by imitation

A social phenomenon seen among adolescents is suicide contagion. Several studies have shown that when one teenager takes his or her life, several more may follow (Gould and Kramer 2001; Poijula *et al.* 2001). Key factors in imitative suicidal behaviour are identification with a victim by age, sex and location. Influences such as economic status, attitudes toward suicide and problem-solving abilities also affect imitative behaviour (Berman 1988).

Today, suicide by imitation seems to be influenced, in part, by its portrayal through mass media (Phillips and Carstensen 1986; Schmidtke and Hafner 1988; Goldney 1989). Coverage of celebrity suicide has been shown to unintentionally encourage suicide. This effect has been labelled 'contagious suicide' or forming a suicide cluster, and has been hypothesised to be caused by a reduction in the individual's resistance to committing the act, the need for attention, or a misguided attempt to find identification and connection with the dead celebrity (Parris 2006). However, mass media's influence can be minimised by avoiding sensationalised reports of suicide that supply details as to the methods used (Jobes *et al.* 1996).

Risk and protective factors for suicidal behaviour

There are many risk and protective factors identified in the literature in relation to suicide and suicidal behaviour. Murray and Hauenstein (2008) and the Registered Nurses' Association of Ontario (RNAO) (2008) have summarised these (see Boxes 6.2, 6.3 and 6.4). It is vital that the presence of risk and protective factors are noted in the patient's clinical notes as part of the risk assessment.

Box 6.2 Risk factors. (Data reproduced with permission from Registered Nurses' Association of Ontario (2008) *Assessment and Care of Adults at Risk of Suicidal Ideation and Behaviour*, Toronto, Canada, and from Murray, B.L. and Hauenstein, E.J. (2008) Self harm and suicide behaviour: children, adolescents and adults. In: *Psychiatric Nursing for Canadian Practice* (eds W. Austin & M.A. Boyd), pp.898–922, copyright 2008 with permission of Lippincott Williams & Wilkins.)

- Demographic or social factors
- Being an older adult
- Being male
- Poverty
- Being Aboriginal
- White race (APA 2003)
- Gay, lesbian or bisexual orientation – assoc. with attempts (APA 2003)
- Being single (widow>divorced>separated>single)
- Social isolation, including new or worsening estrangement, and rural location
- Economic or occupational stress, loss, or humiliation
- New incarceration
- History of gambling
- Easy access to firearms

Box 6.3 Clinical factors. (Data reproduced with permission from Registered Nurses' Association of Ontario (2008) *Assessment and Care of Adults at Risk of Suicidal Ideation and Behaviour,* Toronto, Canada, and from Murray, B.L. and Hauenstein, E.J. (2008) Self harm and suicide behaviour: children, adolescents and adults. In: *Psychiatric Nursing for Canadian Practice* (eds W. Austin & M.A. Boyd), pp.898–922, copyright 2008 with permission of Lippincott Williams & Wilkins.)

- Past and current major psychiatric illness, including bipolar, schizophrenia and major depressive disorder
- Personality disorder (borderline, narcissistic, antisocial)
- Impulsive or violent traits by history
- Current medical illness
- Family history of suicide
- Previous suicide attempts or other self-injurious or impulsive acts
- Current anger, agitation, or constricted preoccupation
- Current abuse of alcohol or drugs
- Easy access to lethal toxins (including prescribed medication)
- Formulated plan, preparations for death or suicide note
- Low ambivalence about dying vs. living
- Childhood trauma (sexual abuse, physical abuse) (APA 2003, p.25)
- Suicidal ideas (current or previous)
- Suicidal intent (APA 2003)
- Hopelessness (APA 2003)
- Severe or unremitting anxiety (APA 2003)
- Panic attacks (APA 2003)
- Impulsiveness (APA 2003)
- Aggression (APA 2003)

Box 6.4   Precipitants and protective factors. (Data reproduced with permission from Registered Nurses' Association of Ontario (2008) *Assessment and Care of Adults at Risk of Suicidal Ideation and Behaviour*, Toronto, Canada, and from Murray, B.L. and Hauenstein, E.J. (2008) Self harm and suicide behaviour: children, adolescents and adults. In: *Psychiatric Nursing for Canadian Practice* (eds W. Austin & M.A. Boyd), pp.898–922, copyright 2008 with permission of Lippincott Williams & Wilkins.)

Precipitants

- Recent stressors (especially losses of emotional, social, physical, or financial security)

Protective factors

- Intact social supports
- Active religious affiliation or faith (may also be a risk factor if shame/guilt about behaviour is involved)
- Marriage and presence of dependent children
- Ongoing supportive relationship with a caregiver
- Positive therapeutic relationship (APA 2003)
- Absence of depression or substance abuse
- Access to medical and mental health resources
- Impulse control
- Proven problem-solving and coping skills
- Pregnancy (APA 2003)
- Life satisfaction (APA 2003)
- Relief about not completing suicide (NZGG 2003)
- Sense of 'unfinished business' (NZGG 2003)
- Good self-esteem, self-confidence (NZGG 2003)
- Awareness of significant others about their suicidal thoughts (NZGG 2003)

Risk to self in the context of the determinants of health (WHO)

Age

Older adults are at a higher risk of attempting suicide compared to other age groups (Gunnell and Middelton 2003). This may be because older adults give few warning signs, use highly planned self-destructive acts and have more determination in achieving their outcome (Conwell *et al.* 1998). In the US in 2004, of every 100,000 people aged 65 and older, 14.3 died by suicide. This figure is higher than the national average of 10.9 suicides per 100,000 people in the general population (National Institute of Mental Health 2005). Non-Hispanic white men aged 85 or older had an even higher rate, with 17.8 suicide deaths per 100,000. Between 1999 and 2004, suicide rates rose by 20% for those aged 45–54 (Center for Disease Control and Prevention (CDC) 2005). In 2004 there were 16.6 completed suicides per 100,000 people in this age group. The rates have not been that high since 1982. In contrast, the suicide rate for people in their twenties rose by only 1%. However, in 2004 suicide was the third leading cause of death in children aged 10–14 (1.3/100,000), adolescents aged 15–19 (8.2/100,000) and young adults (12.5/100,000).

In the UK in 2004, deaths were examined by three age groups. Suicide in older adults aged 75 and older peaked in the early 1990s but has continued to decrease, yet the rate remains the highest of all age groups (Brock *et al.* 2006). The rate for young men (15–44 years old), after an initial stability from 1991, increased by over a fifth between 1997 and 1998, and it was this age group that had the highest male suicide rate from 1998 onwards. For women, up to the mid-1990s, suicide rates decreased in older adults aged 45–74 and 75 and over and slightly increased in young adults (15–44 years old). However, the rate has since stabilised in all age groups and older women aged 75 and over had the highest suicide rate across most of the period.

In 2006 the rates of completed suicide in the UK were as follows:

- for women, 4.4 (15–44 years old), 6.6 (45–74 years old) and 4.5 (75 years old and over) per 100,000;
- for men, 17.7 (15–44 years old), 17.3 (45–74 years old) and 14.9 (75 years old and over) per 100,000.

Self-neglect is also something that one commonly associates with older age. Self-neglect refers to the behaviour of an older person that rejects all domestic comfort and places his or her health or safety at risk (Hwalek 1996). In the elderly self-neglect is due to dementia, cognitive impairment and psychiatric disorder, which results in a limited capacity to engage in self-care actions (Lauder 1998). This is discussed further in the section on self-neglect. Age is also known to be associated with vulnerability and this is more fully discussed in the vulnerability section.

Culture

Culture includes the values, beliefs, attitudes, goals and/or social forms of a particular racial, religious, social or organisational group. Culture may influence thoughts, feelings and attitudes about suicide and self-harm behaviour. Both the client and nurse bring their own culturally derived attitudes, values and beliefs to the therapeutic relationship. As such, culture can greatly impact on how issues of mental health, suicide and death are discussed and addressed in the context of this relationship (RNAO 2008).

Culture may also influence attitudes and behaviour related to self-neglect and vulnerability.

Gender

The rate of suicide worldwide for men was reported as 18.4 per 100,000 in 2000, as opposed to 5.2 for women. It is speculated that the difference in rates of completed suicide may be due to women having a decreased intent to die and the use of less lethal or violent means (Tondo and Baldessarini 2001; WHO 2002).

United Kingdom

The rate of male suicide was over 50% higher in Scotland than the overall rate in the UK from 2002–2004; the rates in Wales and Northern Ireland were also higher than the overall rate of suicide in the UK during this period (Brock *et al.* 2006). Women in Scotland completed suicide at a rate nearly double that of women in England and Wales (10.3 suicides per 100,000 population in Scotland, compared to 5.3 and 5.8 in England and Wales respectively) and was over twice that for Northern Ireland (4.8 per 100,000 population) (Brock *et al.* 2006).

Canada

According to the Public Health Agency of Canada (2000), suicide is the second leading cause of death for males aged 10–34, and the fourth leading cause of death for males aged 35–54; it is the seventh leading cause of death for all ages of males. In comparison, the agency reports that suicide is the second leading cause of death for women aged 15–19, the third leading cause of death for women aged 20–34 and the fourth leading cause of death for women aged 35–54. However, suicide is not in the top 10 for causes of death in Canadian women overall. In 2002, 2,849 men died of intentional self-harm as compared to 799 women; a ratio of 3.5:1. However, women are four times more likely to attempt suicide than are men (Health Canada 2002). Men are 4.5 times more likely to use firearms and women are twice as likely to die by poisoning.

Self-neglect and vulnerability

Gender has been found to be associated with vulnerability. For instance, early maturing girls are more vulnerable to prior psychological problems, deviant peer pressures and fathers' hostile feelings when compared to on-time and late-maturing peers (Ge *et al.* 1996). There is more discussion of this in the vulnerability section. Self-neglect can occur in both genders. Whilst studies have found one gender (males) to be more predictive in their model (Abrams *et al.* 2002), it is highly likely that many confounding variables will be affecting any relationship.

Sexual orientation

'In recent years, sexual orientation as a risk factor for suicide has been highly debated. Russell and Joyner (2001) point to the common belief that having to deal with the stigma of homosexuality may lead gay men and women to depression or even suicide. During adolescence, when the major focus of a youth's life is on peers and sexuality, a gay youth's search for self identity may heighten depression and suicidal behaviour (Rotheram-Borus and Fernandez 1995). 'Coming out' has also been identified as a risk factor in terms of the reactions of others, particularly peers and family. Acknowledging one's sexual orientation at an early age or never disclosing one's sexual orientation can put gay, lesbian, bisexual and transgender (GLBT) youth at a higher risk of suicide (Remafedi et al. 1991). Someone who comes out at an early age is at an increased risk for harassment and assaults, while someone who does not feel safe enough to disclose their sexual orientation may feel extremely isolated (Morrison and L'Heureux 2001). In both cases, there is a feeling of helplessness, hopelessness, powerlessness and isolation, which, regardless of sexual orientation, are feelings that increase the risk of depression and suicide (Beck et al. 1985). GLBT youth are also at a higher risk of suicide if they self-present with high levels of gender nonconformity (Remafedi et al. 1991), report high levels of intrapsychic conflict regarding their sexual orientation (Savin-Williams 1990) or report sexual abuse (Gibson 1994). It is important to note that the risk factors associated with being GLBT are in addition to those common to all ages and sexual orientations' (Murray and Hauenstein 2008, p.903).

This evidence also suggests that one's sexual orientation can significantly affect vulnerability.

Genetics/biological factors

The heritability of suicide is debatable. Twin and adoption studies have also pointed to a possible genetic factor associated with suicidal or self-destructive behaviour, independent of the risk of developing a mood disorder (Parris 2006). Genetic models have estimated that the risk of inheriting an inclination to commit suicide is approximately 45% (Statham *et al.* 1998). Having an identical twin who had made a serious suicide attempt was associated with a 10-fold increase in risk of making such an attempt, a significantly stronger association than that observed in the case of fraternal twin pairs. Twin studies have shown a higher rate of suicide attempts between monozygotic (MZ) twins than dizygotic (DZ) twins, suggesting that genetics are an important factor when examining precipitating factors. In a review of over 20 studies, Baldessarini and Hennen (2004) showed a wide range in the influence of genetics on attempted suicide. One study showed no difference in the likelihood of one twin attempting suicide if the other had, whether they were MZ or DZ twins. However, the majority of studies showed an increased risk of between a four-fold chance and a 175-fold chance of an MZ twin attempting suicide if the other twin had.

> *'Qin et al. (2003) showed that suicidal behaviour in one monozygotic twin increased the risk 11-fold for suicidal behaviour in the co-twin. Another study showed that a serious attempt by one twin increased the risk in a dizygotic co-twin more than twofold and in a monozygotic co-twin almost fourfold (Statham et al. 1998). In this study, genetic factors alone accounted for about half the increased risk for suicidal behaviour. Among adolescent female twins, genetic factors played a part in 35% of suicide attempts (Glowinski et al. 2001). Adoption studies have shown that among adults who experience mood disorders and were adopted as children, the suicide rate among the biologic relatives of the adoptees is much higher than the rate among the adoptive relatives'* (Murray and Hauenstein 2008, p.905).

This suggests that if a person inherits a predisposition towards impulsive and violent behaviour, the risk of committing suicide inevitably goes up (Parris 2006).

Adoption studies have shown that genetic factors, rather than familial environmental factors, are the major determinants of familial concordance for suicidal behaviour. Schulsinger *et al.* (1979) reported a higher incidence of suicide in the biological relatives of adopted suicide victims compared with the biological relatives of matched, non-suicide controls. Baldessarini and Hennen's (2004) review similarly showed that the risk of someone who was adopted attempting suicide was between three and six times greater if they had a first-degree relative attempt suicide.

These studies suggest that genetic factors may be partly responsible for suicide attempts but do not allow definite conclusions to be drawn about the degree to which genetics plays a role nor the relative importance of environmental influences and psychiatric disorders (Statham *et al.* 1998). However, these authors also note that controlling for psychiatric history and for other psychosocial variables, an MZ co-twin's history of suicidal thoughts and behaviour remained a powerful predictor of increased risk of attempted suicide.

Social support networks, social environment and healthy child development

Children's families are central to their healthy development. They provide the early love, stimulation and security that prepare them to enter into other relationships and other environments (Health Canada 1994). However, not all children and adolescents grow up in a safe, loving environment. Many experience and are exposed to abuse, neglect and adverse circumstances. Those who are exposed to multiple adversity and lack meaningful attachments during childhood and adolescence are at an elevated risk of suicide (DeWilde *et al.* 1992). However, there have been few studies investigating the role that childhood adversities, negative life events and interpersonal difficulties may play in the development of suicidal behaviour (Kushner and Sterk 2005). Therefore, the link between adverse life experiences and suicidal ideation and behaviour remains somewhat unknown (Kienhorst *et al.* 1995; Wagner 1997). That said there is research that points to an association between interpersonal relationships and risk of suicide.

Durkheim linked modern urban life to increased alienation and strained gender roles which he believed had negative health consequences, evidenced by increased suicide rates (Gould *et al.* 1996), and viewed suicide, in part, as a consequence of the deterioration of social and familial bonds (Fergusson *et al.* 2000). More recently, case-control and longitudinal studies (Silove *et al.* 1987; Reinherz *et al.* 1995) have indicated that adversities such as poor family relationships and stressful life events are associated with suicidal behaviour.

Kushner and Sterk (2005) suggest that interpersonal conflict may also play a role in predicting suicidal behaviour during adulthood. Their findings are consistent with past research which indicates that stressful life events may be associated with childhood adversities and suicidal behaviour during adolescence or early adulthood. Youths who experience numerous adversities during childhood and adolescence are at a particularly elevated risk of suicide.

Developmental theorists suggest there is a correlation between negative life events and interpersonal difficulties, which could be used in determining whether childhood adversities contribute to the onset of suicidal behaviour. Kushner and Sterk's (2005) findings are consistent with previous studies showing that the disruption of interpersonal relationships is a predominant risk factor for suicide. Children who experience high levels of maladaptive parenting, such as affectionless and/or over-protective parenting, are also at a high risk of suicide (Goldney 1985; Adam *et al.* 1994; Wagner and Cohen 1994). Furthermore, those who experience child abuse may have difficulty in developing social skills that are essential for the maintenance of healthy relationships with peers and adults. Without the required skill, individuals can develop maladaptive interpersonal coping behaviour which may contribute to the onset of despair, hopelessness and suicidal behaviour (Kushner and Sterk 2005).

Warning signs or invitations to help

Warning signs or invitations to help are usually of two types:

- stressful events involving feelings of loss;
- reactions to events and life circumstances (Ramsay *et al.* 2004).

A reaction to loss and stressful events is highly individualised. Most people are able to cope with stressors in their lives without turning to suicide. This is accomplished through both internal resources (resilience, adaptability, coping strategies) and external supports (friends, families, community services). Stress becomes distress when these resources are overwhelmed, whether gradually or catastrophically (Ramsay *et al.* 2004). Thoughts of suicide may arise if the stress is viewed as never-ending, intolerable or inescapable and suicidal behaviour becomes more likely when something happens or may happen that produces a sense of overwhelming loss (Ramsay *et al.* 2004). However, the intensity of a stressor or event, a large number of stressors or persistent stress do not necessarily lead to suicidal behaviour. A particular event may be a precipitating factor, a trigger that is just one last event, loss or stressor to deal with and is often the 'straw that broke the camel's back', building on many other stressful events or losses. Suicidal behaviour is usually associated with an accumulation of loss.

People who experience loss or stress usually talk about the loss and give warning signs or invitations to help. It is important for mental health nurses to be cognisant of possible stressors or loss in their patients' lives in order to explore their patients' personal feelings and perception of the loss. A person's thoughts, feelings, behaviours and/or physical functioning may each reveal or reflect the person's distress and give indications of an invitation to help (Ramsay *et al.* 2004).

The framework in Box 6.5 may be used to organise observations based on seeing, hearing and sensing. It also includes potentially stressful situations that may lead someone to consider suicide. Case study 1 in Box 6.6 provides an example of how some of these principles apply.

Box 6.5 Invitations to help. (Reproduced from Ramsay, R.F, Yanney, B.L., Lang, W.A. & Kinzel, T. (2004) *Suicide Intervention Handbook*, copyright 2004 with permission of Living Works Education Inc.)

Learn about SITUATIONS:

- Relationship problems
- Work problems/failing grades
- Trouble with the law
- Recent suicide and violence, much publicised

Almost anything depending upon how the person feels about it

Ask about PHYSICAL CHANGES:

- Lack of interest/pleasure in all things
- Lack of physical energy
- Disturbed sleep
- Change/loss of sexual interest
- Change/loss of appetite/weight
- Physical health complaints

Observe BEHAVIOURS:

- Crying
- Emotional outbursts
- Alcohol/drug misuse
- Recklessness
- Fighting/law breaking
- Withdrawal
- Dropping out
- Prior suicidal behavior
- Putting affairs in order

Listen for THOUGHTS:

- Escape
- No future
- Guilty
- Alone
- Damaged
- Helpless
- Preoccupied
- Talk of suicide or death
- Planning for suicide

Sense FEELINGS:

- Desperate
- Angry
- Sad
- Ashamed
- Worthless
- Lonely
- Disconnected
- Hopeless

Box 6.6   Case study: Mrs Davidson.

Situation

You are caring for Mrs Davidson who has been admitted with a primary diagnosis of depression and a secondary diagnosis of cancer of the breast. She is a widow and lives alone. Although she has three adult children, they do not live in the same city as her. As you are doing her morning care she indicates that life is not worth living any more and her children would be 'better off if she passed on as they would receive the benefits of her life insurance policy'.

Nurse's interpretation

The nurse recognises that a terminal diagnosis and a depressive response may lead to feelings of suicide. The nurse is aware that Mrs Davidson lives alone and does not have any children living nearby. Although Mrs Davidson does not directly state that she is suicidal, the nurse picks up on the risk factors, the lack of protective factors and the possible warning signs or invitations to help.

Nurse's action

The nurse takes Mrs Davidson's statement as serious and initiates a comprehensive assessment of risk including an exploration of Mrs Davidson's perspective of her stressors and life situation. The nurse establishes a therapeutic relationship and actively listens as Mrs Davidson tells her story. The nurse plans interventions based on the assessment of risk and evaluates their outcomes.

Vulnerability

Certain populations are more vulnerable and at-risk of abuse than others. Children are more vulnerable than adults, girls and women are more vulnerable than males, and people with disabilities are more vulnerable than the non-disabled. The high prevalence of sexual abuse among children and adults with developmental disabilities has been widely documented (Sobsey and Varnhagen 1988, 1989, 1991; MacDonald 1994; Sobsey 1994; Barrett *et al.* 1997). Youths with developmental disabilities are particularly vulnerable to trauma and abuse (physical, emotional and sexual) and having a disability in itself can be traumatic (Sinason 1992). Trauma and abuse can also be a result of not only the immediate environment but also community and professional systems and the wider systems such as political and legal (Halliday and Mackrell 1998).

Prevalence data indicate that 4–10% of people with developmental disabilities display self-harm behaviour (Halliday and Mackrell 1998), and approximately 90% of people who self-harm have severe or profound learning disabilities (Oliver *et al.* 1987). Prevalence rates are also generally higher for:

- males than females;
- people who are non-verbal or have problems with communication;
- people with sensory impairment;
- people with environmental disadvantages;
- those with a dual-diagnosis of developmental disability and mental illness

(Borthwick-Duffy 1994; Oliver 1995; Gates 2000).

Self-harm behaviour (SHB) may be the manifestation of a genetic syndrome (Plomin *et al.* 1994; Gates 2000; Schroeder *et al.* 2001); however, the presence of a genetic syndrome alone is not always sufficient to cause SHB. It is usually more accepted that a combined effect of developmental disability and environment cause SHB in subjects with specific genetic disorders (Shoumitro 1996). SHB may also be manifested in the context of:

- neurological disorders, for example, Tourette Syndrome (Robertson *et al.* 1989);
- psychiatric disorders;
- a wide range of clinical symptoms and conditions (Bodfish 1999);
- developmental disorders such as mental retardation and autism (Lewis and Bodfish 1998).

Suicidal behaviours are often related to issues surrounding sexual abuse.

Both the Roeher Institute at York University and the University of Alberta Abuse and Disability Project have conducted extensive research in the area of violence and abuse in the lives of people with disabilities. In 1992 the Roeher Institute indicated that 39–68% of girls with a mental handicap and 16–30% of boys with a mental handicap will be sexually abused before the age of 18. They also stated that it is alarmingly probable that a person with a mental handicap approaching adulthood will already have experienced some form of sexual abuse. Dick Sobsey, a member of the University of Alberta Abuse and Disability Project, confirmed these findings in 1994. He also stated that most people with disabilities will experience some form of sexual assault or abuse and people who have some level of intellectual impairment are at the highest risk of abuse.

Among adults with developmental disabilities, as many as 83% of females and 32% of males are the victims of sexual assault (Johnson and Sigler 2000). Males with disabilities are twice as likely as males without disabilities to be sexually abused in their lifetime (Statistics Canada 1994). The abuse of people with disabilities is often invisible due to the many barriers to disclosure (e.g. fear, economic dependence, isolation, lack of access to supports and credibility issues), and when it is identified it is often unreported (The Peoples Law School 2004). Reports are usually limited to serious instances and verbal and psychological abuses, and cases of restraint and control are almost never reported (Sobsey 1994). It is estimated that only 3% of sexual abuse cases involving people with developmental disabilities are ever reported (Lawlink 2003).

The profile of the sexual abuse of people with developmental disabilities has specific differences compared to sexual abuse and the general population. In children with disabilities, the perpetrators of sexual abuse are similar to non-disabled children, with acquaintances and family members making up the highest group. However, in adolescence, service providers become the highest group of perpetrators, especially where the person has a severe disability. Other service users also constitute a significant group for adults (Westcott and Jones 1999). Also people with developmental disabilities are less likely to escape the abuse because of their dependence on caregivers and, sometimes, limited communication. Perpetrators do gravitate to working in such places where there is access and opportunity to abuse these clients with less likelihood of detection (Lawlink 2003).

Self-neglect

The typical image of self-neglect, that of poor personal hygiene, an unkempt household and poor health, is not unfamiliar to most health professionals. The client with self-neglect is usually portrayed as being elderly and having some degree of dementia or depression. The medical model has described self-neglect as being multifaceted involving an inability or refusal to care for one's own health, social needs, nutrition and hygiene (Lachs *et al.* 1996) with the assumption that there is an underlying medical condition in need of treatment (Lauder 1998). In other words, the medical model proposes that those with a mental illness do not have the capacity to care or remember to care for themselves (Lauder 1998).

It has been suggested that self-neglect exists on a continuum from poor self-grooming to neglect that promotes disease and could lead to death (Rathbone-McCuan and Bricker-Jenkins 1992). However, self-neglect is no longer thought of as a predetermined effect of dementia or depression. Johnson and Adams (1996) suggest that in a client without mental illness, self-neglect may be a choice rather than an inevitability. Lauder (1998) supports this notion, stating that the presence of a mental illness does not predispose an individual to self-neglect nor does self-neglect indicate a mental illness. Therefore, the identification and diagnosis of self-neglect may not be as cut and dried as the medical model suggests.

While there is evidence that those with mental illness such as depression and dementia engage in self-neglect and while it is possible that clients have many life problems that render self-care less important, it cannot be denied that the interpretation of self-neglect can be coloured by the personal and professional beliefs of healthcare professionals regarding adequate self-care (Lauder 1998). Therefore, in identifying and diagnosing self-neglect, healthcare professionals must be careful that their assessment is not constructed on value-laden assumptions of what determines adequate self-care. Rather, self-care must be understood within the context that the client exists, questioning whether there is an underlying medical condition manifested in self-neglect or whether it is the choice of the client regarding his or her level of self-care, which we perhaps consider to be neglect because it does not meet with our idea of adequate care as health professionals.

ADPIE (Assessment, Diagnosis, Plan, Intervention, Evaluation)

Psychiatric mental health nursing practice standards define the nursing process within the context of five standards of care (assessment, diagnosis, plan/outcome, intervention(s) and evaluation). The purpose of assessment is to identify and clearly articulate specific problems in the individual's life that are causing physical or mental disequilibrium or harm. The assessment may be based on observation, interviews, history taking, physical examination and mental status. A nursing diagnosis provides the basis for the selection of nursing interventions chosen to achieve outcomes for which the nurse is accountable (North American Nursing Diagnosis Association International (NANDA) 2006). The plan affects the goals and aids in the continuity of care for the client. Interventions are the actions nurses take to carry out the nursing measures identified in the care plan to achieve the expected outcome criteria. Evaluation is often the most neglected part of the nursing process. Ideally, evaluation should be part of each phase in the process.

Although the discussion that follows in relation to ADPIE is in the context of suicidal behaviour, the principles may also be applied to vulnerable individuals and those at risk of self-neglect .

Assessment

'Risk to self is seriously underreported and often unrecognized by health care professionals. Estimates are that approximately 40% of people who complete suicide have visited a health care provider within 1 to 6 months of a suicide attempt (Foster et al. 1999, Link et al. 1999). Nurses can play important roles in suicide prevention because they practice in diverse health care settings and thus work with various groups of patients. Acutely suicidal behaviour is a true psychiatric emergency. Nurses must act immediately and vigorously to prevent the patient's death' (Murray and Hauenstein 2008, p.909).

A comprehensive suicide assessment is always considered a priority. Taking the time to engage and connect with the patient prior to the assessment is crucial (Murray 2003). As a nurse it is important to integrate an assessment process that delineates:

- stressors;
- symptoms;
- prior suicidal behaviour;
- current plan;
- available identified resources and support

(Ramsay *et al.* 1994).

Nursing interventions based on a comprehensive assessment of risk provide a holistic approach to nursing care of the suicidal patient. The process of risk assessment will be discussed, followed by a discussion of nursing diagnosis, interventions and evaluation.

Comprehensive assessment of risk to self

'A model developed by the first author (B.L.M.) integrates a number of theories to establish a comprehensive assessment of risk. The model emphasizes an approach that views the patient in context of their family, their social world and the broader community (Murray and Wright 2006). It encourages engagement and the development of a connectedness with the client and their family using the language of a Brief Solutions and Family Therapy approach (Berg 1994, Corcoran 1998, DeShazer 1988, Eggert and Thompson 2002, Minuchin and Fishman 1981, O'Hanlon and Werner-Davis 1989) emphasizing the power and resiliency of families as key components for change and resolution. An intergenerational perspective and use of the genogram (deGraaf 1998, McGoldrick 1992) are also an integral part of the approach. This perspective recognizes family patterns over time and traces the history of abuse, alcoholism, trauma and loss (Maine et al. 2001, Gould and Kramer 2001). Recognition of developmental factors that contribute to individual and family struggles, and family interactional patterns and boundaries also assists in providing a broad and complete assessment' (Murray and Hauenstein 2008, pp.909–910).

'Applied Suicide Intervention Skills Training (ASIST)/Living Works Inc. (Ramsay et al. 1994) provides the framework for risk assessment, emphasizing assessment of stressors, symptoms, prior suicidal behaviour, current plan, and resources and support. An overall Rogerian approach (Rogers 1980) guides the interactions with the patient and their family with a non-blaming, non-judgmental, and unconditional positive regard approach to understand and process what the suicidal ideation or behaviour is really about. Integration of the model also assists

in understanding the onset, the purpose, the maintenance, and the escalation of the suicidal behaviour and assesses specific risk factors related to the self-harm behaviour' (Murray and Hauenstein 2008, p.910).

Stressors

'A comprehensive assessment of stressors is vital to guide appropriate interventions. Assessment includes collection of adequate data to provide a clear picture of the patient's life and relevant stressors. As much as possible, the patient's perspective of their stressors, and their life situations should be explored. This includes a good understanding of their family, peers, and social relationships as well as workplace issues. Past loss issues need to be explored with the patient to identify any possible precipitating factors related to change or loss. It is also important to discuss issues of abuse and to be aware that these issues must be approached with the appropriate degree of sensitivity' (Murray and Hauenstein 2008, p.910).

Symptoms

'Symptoms may be explored in context of a depression assessment keeping in mind the broad spectrum of depressive symptoms ranging from isolating or withdrawing from friends and family, sleep and eating disturbances, and/or not enjoying or participating in activities or functions that were enjoyed in the past, to acting out/risky behaviour such as rebellion, non-compliance, and/or drugs or alcohol use (Ramsay et al. 1994)' (Murray and Hauenstein 2008, p.910).

Many useful screens for depressive symptoms are available. The Center for Epidemiological Studies Depression Scale (CES-D) (Radloff 1977) is a 20-item self-report questionnaire that takes less than 10 minutes to complete. Each of the 20 items is a symptom of depression; the patient is asked to report how many days in the last week he or she has experienced the symptom. The range of possible scores is 0 to 60. People with a score above 16 may have major depressive disorder (MDD); those with scores above 25 are probably clinically depressed. Other self-rating or clinician-rated scales include the Zung Self-Rating Depression Scale (Zung 1965) and the Beck Depression Inventory (Beck *et al.* 1961).

'In 1997, Beck revised the Scale for Suicide Ideation (Beck et al. 1997, Beck et al. 1979a) to include only eight items, and renamed it the Suicide Intent Scale. This scale is short and useful in determining whether a patient has a strong intent to die. The nurse or another experienced professional should assess the patient for other psychiatric disorders, especially those most commonly associated with suicidal behaviour. E.g. MDD, panic disorder, severe anxiety disorder,

schizophrenia, substance abuse, borderline personality disorder, and antisocial personality disorder (Brieger et al. 2002, Catallozzi et al. 2001, Preuss et al. 2002, Prigerson and Slimack 1999, Radomsky et al. 1999)' (Murray and Hauenstein 2008, p.911).

'Severity of MDD is associated with a greater likelihood of suicide completion (Alexopoulos et al. 1999, Grant and Hasin 1999). For adolescents, a key question is whether any family member has attempted or completed suicide (Cerel et al. 1999, Klimes-Dougan et al. 1999, McKeown et al. 1998). Alcoholism is another prominent factor in suicide. Patients with alcoholism account for 25% of completed suicides (Berglund and Ojehagen 1998)' (Murray and Hauenstein 2008, p.911).

Prior self-harm behaviour

'Assessing the context of each act of prior self-harm behaviour begins to paint a picture of motivation behind the behaviour. Exploration of prior behaviour also gives a message of interest and concern on the part of the health professional and a non-blaming, non-judgmental approach allows further exploration and understanding of the patient's situation as they begin to trust the therapeutic relationship' (Murray and Hauenstein 2008, p.911).

Knowledge of others' self-harm behaviour

'Assessment also includes exploration of self-harm behaviour that has been observed by the patient. Self-harm behaviour can be imitative especially if it is interpreted as a way of coping with frustration and anger or a way of punishing self or others (Rew et al. 2001). Depending on the reaction of others, people may misunderstand self-harm behaviour as an acceptable way to cope with a difficult or intolerable life' (Murray and Hauenstein 2008, p.911).

Others' reaction to self-harm behaviour

'Others' reaction of self-harm behaviour needs to be explored. Whether or not the response was the predicted and desired response is also important. Expected or desired responses must be explored to help patients meet their needs, wants, and desires in more acceptable and appropriate ways' (Murray and Hauenstein 2008, p.911).

Current plan

'A suicide requires intent, a plan, knowledge of how to carry out the act, and few obstacles to completing it. Patients who complete suicide have developed a

workable method of killing themselves. They are less likely to have young children or other immediate responsibilities and may not be concerned with religious prohibitions on the act. The relationship between the availability of a method of suicide and suicide completion is strong (Cantor and Baume 1998). It is important to ask if the patient has a current plan for suicide. Further exploration of the plan gives the nurse a more accurate assessment of risks and guides appropriate interventions' (Murray and Hauenstein 2008, p.911).

It is important to use a non-blaming and non-reactionary approach to accomplish an in-depth exploration of the current plan.

'It is also important to recognise that some people will carefully prepare to take their own lives whereas others may impulsively end their lives. The people who are usually impulsive are adolescents, people who abuse alcohol or drugs, or people with personality disorders. Patients with psychoses may also act impulsively to "voices" that direct them to kill themselves. Patients with psychoses are at considerable risk because of their inability to separate psychotic thinking from reality' (Murray and Hauenstein 2008, p.911).

People who have developed a plan and the means to carry it out and who have executed some parts of the plan are serious about their intent to kill themselves.

There is no evidence to suggest that asking a person directly about the topic of suicide will increase the likelihood of suicidal ideation and behaviour (American Psychiatric Association (APA) 2003; New Zealand Guidelines Group (NZGG) 2003; RNAO 2008). According to the APA (2003), *'Asking about suicide is necessary and will not lead the person to suicide'* (p.19). An assessment specific to factors related to suicide helps to uncover the purpose and meaning behind any suicidal ideation and behaviour, thereby informing the development of appropriate and meaningful interventions (Murray and Hauenstein 2008).

Resources and support

'Lack of resources and support may put patients at the greatest risk for self-harm behaviour. It is also important to explore supportive people in the patient's life, as identified by them' (Murray and Hauenstein 2008, p.911).

Supportive people are those to whom patients are comfortable communicating their struggles and difficulties. Most victims of suicide feel socially isolated. They generally cannot name anyone in their immediate environment who is supportive or with whom they can stay while they are acutely suicidal. They often wish to be alone or are unwilling to ask anyone for help.

*'Interest in the patient's life and attention received during a thorough assess-
ment is also therapeutic and provides connectedness and engagement with the
patient and their family. This connectedness provides the therapeutic environment necessary to engage the patient and their family in meaningful change'*
(Jobes 2000, cited in Murray and Hauenstein 2008, p.911).

This comprehensive analysis provides a clear picture of the self-harm
behaviour and guides possible interventions (see Box 6.7 for suggested questions to guide a comprehensive assessment of risk). In addition it is useful
to include aspects of a psychiatric assessment, for example:

- past psychiatric history;
- past medical history;
- current and past medications;
- drug allergies.

It is also useful to conduct a mental status examination, for instance of
the following:

- appearance;
- behaviour;
- attitude;
- affect;
- mood;
- psychomotor activity;
- speech;
- thought content and process;
- perception;
- orientation;
- insight;
- judgment;
- cognition.

Box 6.7 Questions to guide a comprehensive assessment of risk. (Reproduced
from Murray, B.L. & Hauenstein, E.J. (2008) Self harm and suicide behaviour:
children, adolescents and adults. In: *Psychiatric Nursing for Canadian Practice*
(eds W. Austin & M.A. Boyd), pp. 898–922, copyright 2008 with permission of
Lippincott Williams & Wilkins.)

The most successful approach is to ask open-ended questions and explore further
with curious questions.

Stressors
What is troubling you most at the moment?

- Explore with curious questions in terms of all areas of the patient's life.
- Explore each area, asking the patient to tell you more.

The idea is to get a clear picture of the patient's life situation and his or her presenting stressors as he/she perceives them.

Symptoms
Can you tell me about your sleep patterns?

- Explore using curious questions:
  - Are you having difficulty sleeping?
  - Do you want to stay in bed and sleep through the day?

Can you tell me about your eating habits?

- Explore using curious questions:
  - Have you lost your appetite?
  - Do you eat in an attempt to cope with difficulties?

What do you do for enjoyment?

- Explore with curious questions:
  - Do you find you no longer enjoy activities you thought were enjoyable?
  - How often do you use drugs or alcohol to cope?

Prior behaviour
Have you ever thought of harming yourself?

- Explore with curious questions:
  - Can you tell me about that? (time, place, situation, feelings, meaning)
  - What was the self-harm about?
  - What happened?
  - What did you expect to happen?
  - What did you want to happen?

Current plan
Do you have a plan at the moment to harm yourself?

- Explore with curious questions:
  - What would you do?
  - Do you have access to the pills? (other methods)
  - Have you picked a specific day or time?

Resources and support
Do you have someone you recognise as supportive?

- Explore with curious questions:
  - Who can you talk to about your concerns?
  - Who can you confide in?
  - Offer suggestions of a number of people the patient may not have thought of (e.g. parent's friend, colleague, clergy, coach, etc.).

Diagnosis

The primary factor in diagnosis is the recognition of the risk of suicide or self-harm behaviour. Examples of possible nursing diagnosis would include:

- risk of self harm and/or life-threatening injury;
- risk of self-directed violence;
- impaired social interaction;
- ineffective coping;
- interrupted family processes;
- ineffective health maintenance.

Examples of related diagnosis for self-neglect and vulnerability would include:

- self-care deficit related to a psychological disability due to impaired self worth, or substance abuse, or age or mental illness;
- self-care deficit related to vulnerability due to cognitive impairment, or age, or gender or sexual orientation.

Plan

It is important to develop a plan for safety and care determined by the outcome of the risk to self assessment. The care plan should reflect the risk factors specific to the individual, expected outcomes (immediate, stabilisation and community), nursing interventions and the rationale for each intervention. Before the patient's release, a specific, concrete plan for outpatient care must be in place. The care plan includes scheduling an appointment for outpatient care, providing for continuing medication until the first outpatient treatment visit, ensuring post-release contact between the patient and significant other, providing for access to emergency psychiatric care, and arranging the patient's environment so that it provides both structure and safety (Murray and Hauenstein 2008).

Interventions

Establishment of a therapeutic relationship

'Thorough assessment becomes part of the intervention process, as the health professional's genuine interest, concern and exploration begins to establish the trusting relationship that is needed' (Murray and Hauenstein 2008, p.911).

The therapeutic relationship describes the interpersonal process that occurs between the nurse and the client(s), and is based on trust, respect and the advancement of the client's best interest and outcomes (RNAO 2006). The establishment of a therapeutic relationship provides the opportunity for the healthcare professional to foster hope with the suicidal client and to work towards minimising the client's feelings of shame, guilt and stigma that may be associated with suicidality, mental illness and addiction (RNAO 2008). Both APA (2003) and NZGG (2003) guidelines suggest that positive therapeutic relationships have protective effects for suicide.

In addition, there are particular circumstances that may pose challenges to the establishment of a therapeutic relationship. These include:

- a highly agitated, despondent, or paranoid client;
- the nurse's own feelings toward death and suicide;
- issues of transference and counter-transference.

Working through these challenging situations is essential and requires collaboration, mentorship and clinical supervision (RNAO 2008).

Understanding the meaning of the suicidal behaviour

'Understanding the purpose and meaning of the self-harm behaviour facilitates and guides the intervention strategies. It also gives the patient and their family a sense of hope that things can change, that someone understands their situation and is willing to assist them in making the changes that they have identified. If behaviour is understood as a means of communication then interventions will be directed at achieving ends with more acceptable behaviour. Health care professionals are then able to help patients identify what and who needs to change in their environment and also assist in identifying very concrete areas for improvement or change. This empowers the client to address their feelings of hopelessness, helplessness and powerlessness' (Murray and Hauenstein 2008, p.912).

It is important for the mental health nurse to understand the situation from the client's perspective and assist the client in understanding the connection between his or her suicidal behaviour and present and past stressors and issues. Many clients have not made this connection or they may have difficulty making the connection. It is also important to assist the client in developing more effective problem solving and coping skills. Understanding the connection and engaging in more appropriate forms of coping empowers clients to be in control of their situation.

The mental health nurse should take seriously all statements and/or behaviours that indicate either directly or indirectly a risk of suicide or self-harm behaviour. *'Taking seriously'* means to:

- conduct a suicide risk assessment;
- document the assessment;
- discuss the assessment with other members of the client's healthcare team;
- create a plan for safety and care as determined by the outcome of the assessment (RNAO 2008).

Clients may underestimate the lethality of the self-harm behaviour or they may have impulsive behaviour; therefore every episode of self-harm must be assessed for lethality and care needs to be taken that self-harm events are not minimised or trivialised. Suicide cannot always be prevented; however, the nurse has both a legal and ethical responsibility to do whatever is possible to prevent a suicide from occurring.

Safety

It is important for the healthcare professional to assess and manage factors that may impact the physical safety of the client and the interprofessional team. It is always important for the nurse to ensure his or her safety first and this may involve requesting the assistance of other members of the healthcare or safety team. The nurse also needs to be aware of items in the physical environment that may pose a risk of harm. The major deterrent to patients completing suicide in psychiatric hospitals is their engagement in a therapeutic relationship and regular observation by nurses (RNAO 2008).

> *'Maintaining a safe environment includes observing the patient regularly for suicidal behaviour, removing dangerous objects, and providing counselling opportunities for the patient. Part of ensuring patient safety is helping patients to re-establish personal control by including them in decisions about their care and restricting their behaviour only as necessary. It is important for the nurse to have ongoing and effective communication with the patient to allow the patient to disclose and discuss their life situation and the resulting emotions and behaviour'* (Murray and Hauenstein 2008, p.913).

Observation should therefore be utilised to assist the client in feeling cared for and as an opportunity to engage with the client in a therapeutic relationship.

Treatment modalities

It is important for the healthcare professional to be aware of current treatments in order to provide advocacy, referral, monitoring and health teaching interventions, as appropriate.

Psychotherapy

Psychotherapy is a:

> '. . . *treatment method for mental illness in which a mental health professional and a patient discuss problems and feelings to find solutions. Psychotherapy can help individuals change their thinking and behaviour patterns or understanding of how past experience affects current behaviour'* (National Institute of Mental Health 2005).

Psychotherapeutic interventions are most likely to be effective in preventing suicide when they address the specific adversities experienced by each individual. People who are at an elevated risk of suicide may benefit most from clinical interventions that help them to overcome a prolonged history of severe interpersonal difficulties (Leenaars 2004). Psychotherapy is a human exchange. Effective psychotherapy should be person-centred. Person-centred psychotherapy, whether cognitive or otherwise, is derived from the focus on the individual – the individual in his or her entirety, i.e., biological, psychological, sociological and so on. Edwin Shneidman commented on psychotherapy with suicidal patients as follows:

> 'Our treatment, psychotherapy, should address the person's story, not the demographic, nosological categories or this or that fact. It is not what the clinician knows. It is the clinician's understanding of the person's story; each individual's own story. It says, please tell me who you are . . . what hurts' (Leenaars 2004).

Beck (2002) has also developed key concepts regarding suicide and its prevention. His primary finding was the concept of hopelessness, and his studies confirm it as a predictor of eventual suicide. Beck supports brief cognitive therapy treatment for those at high risk of attempting suicide and who may also have significant psychopathology or substance abuse issues. Cognitive processing in suicidal individuals has two features: a high degree of hopelessness and a cognitive deficit or difficulty in solving problems (Beck and Emery 1985). Although the hopelessness accentuates poor problem solving and vice versa, difficulties in coping with life situations can, by themselves, contribute to suicidal potential (Corsini and Wedding 2005).

> 'It is important for nurses to use the hospitalization period to find out what may have precipitated or contributed to the suicidal crisis. Often, the precipitating

factors and how the patient's coping process began to break down are evident. After identifying extreme stressors experienced by the patient, the nurse and patient can help determine ways for the patient to avoid those stressors in the future or, if they cannot be avoided, to manage them more effectively' (Murray and Hauenstein 2008, p.914).

Psychotherapy can also be an important treatment modality during hospitalisation.

'The hospitalization is a good time for the nurse to evaluate the patient's ways of thinking about problems and generating solutions. Some patients, by virtue of their depressive illness or social learning, have an unusually negative view of life. They often think such thoughts as, "I am no good," "Everything I do is useless," "I have no future," or "Nobody has ever liked me, and nobody ever will." Often patients are unable to recognize the connection between their stressors and their suicidal behaviour. Many patients have had very difficult and abusive experiences in their lives and their ability to cope is being threatened. It is important for the nurse to help the patient identify what needs to change in their life, and how that change can come about most effectively. It is also useful to identify who can assist in making the identified changes possible. The prevention of suicidal behaviour is dependent on the patient's belief that they can make changes with the necessary support and resources and there is hope for the future' (Murray and Hauenstein 2008, p.914).

Psychopharmacology

'Psychopharmacology is a subspecialty of pharmacology that includes medications used to affect the brain and behaviours related to psychiatric disorders' (Hegadoren and McCabe Boyd 2008, p.197).

'The objective of medication for suicidal behaviour is to raise serotonin rapidly to a level that reduces suicide risk (Nemeroff et al. 2001). To that end, third-generation and newer antidepressant medications should be used for those who are in imminent danger of harming themselves. These include fluoxetine (Prozac), sertraline (Zoloft), paroxetine (Serzone), bupropion (Wellbutrin), venlafaxine (Effexor), and citalopram (Celexa). These drugs generally are nontoxic and cause few side effects, especially after being taken for 1 to 2 weeks. They often are faster acting than the older drugs, but their onset of action varies. Especially useful are fluoxetine and paroxetine, which may be taken once a day. Sertraline also can be taken once a day, but achieving the proper dose sometimes can be difficult. Patients who take an overdose of these medications have much better outcomes than those who abuse first- and second-generation antidepressants' (Murray and Hauenstein 2008, pp. 913–914).

'*The first- and second-generation antidepressants, including tricyclics and mono-amine oxidase inhibitors, are equally effective for severe depression (Sutherland et al. 2003). However, for those with suicidal behaviour they may not be the best choice. These are highly toxic medications that people with suicidal intent can use to kill themselves. Resuscitation of a patient who has taken large amounts of one of these medications can be difficult because they are cardiotoxic. Medical sequelae may be long term if the patient is saved. The side effects of these early antidepressants may result in the patient stopping the use of prescribed medication while still having suicidal thoughts. The need for laboratory assessment for therapeutic drug levels is another disadvantage of these drugs. Blood monitoring requires the patient's cooperation when his or her motivation may be at its lowest*' (Murray and Hauenstein 2008, p.914).

ECT

ECT can be a life-saving procedure for the acutely suicidal patient or chronically depressed individual. Since there is no evidence for long-term or sustained reduction of suicide risk after an acute course of ECT, close monitoring and additional treatment with psychotropic mediations are usually required during subsequent weeks and months (APA 2003).

Substance abuse treatment

'*Suicidal behaviour is often associated with substance abuse, especially among men. When substance abuse is an issue for the suicidal patient, the abuse must be addressed or inpatient treatment of suicidal behaviour is only palliative, and the danger of the patient repeating a suicidal threat or attempt is high. For men, substance abuse may be the primary psychiatric disorder and depression a side effect of it. For women, depression commonly is the primary psychiatric disorder, and substance abuse results from attempts to medicate the underlying depressive condition*' (Murray and Hauenstein 2008, p.914).

Successful treatment of suicidal behaviour in both men and women requires substance abuse treatment. The nurse should work with the physician and patient to identify a suitable substance abuse treatment programme. The nurse should also be sure that the patient understands the role that alcohol and drugs play in suicidal behaviour.

Evaluation and follow-up

'*The most desirable treatment outcome is the patient's return to the community. Because most hospitalizations for suicidal behaviour are brief, discharge planning must begin immediately after the patient is admitted. The nurse needs to explain to the patient that hospitalization is likely to be short term, and immediately begin to form a partnership with the patient and family to ensure a smooth transition to the community. Partnering means empowering the patient to engage in self-care as soon as possible by helping to provide the tools he or she needs to manage'* (Murray and Hauenstein 2008, pp.915–916).

Important in the process is the evaluation of whether the treatment approaches were effective or deficient and whether the problem was resolved or not. Promotion of realistic self appraisal by the client is also important, with discussion focused on clients' perceptions of their abilities and challenges and reinforcement of the ability of clients to appraise themselves.

'Before discharge, it is ideal for the patient to be able to name people who can act as a support. When supportive people are present, with the patient's permission, the nurse can work with them to begin to develop a network for the patient to rely on to remain safe. It is important for the patient and their supportive family and friends to have a plan to contact another person, either a confidante or a mental health care provider, when they have questions or distressing thoughts or feel unable to manage the situation' (Murray and Hauenstein 2008, p.914)

'Most suicides occur during the first week after discharge, and many happen within the first 24 hours (Appleby et al. 1999a). Before the patient's release, a specific, concrete plan for outpatient care must be in place. The care plan includes scheduling an appointment for outpatient care, providing for continuing medication until the first outpatient treatment visit, ensuring post release contact between the patient and significant other, providing for access to emergency psychiatric care, and arranging the patient's environment so that it provides both structure and safety. In the end, it is the patient, not supporters, who must bear responsibility for his or her safety. The patient who feels connected to but not dependent on significant others will be most likely to maintain safety in the community' (Murray and Hauenstein 2008, p.916).

'Finally, there should be some continuity between inpatient and outpatient care. The nurse must tell the patient specifically how to obtain emergency psychiatric care. He or she should place written instructions near the patient's telephone. It is helpful for the community nurse, in addition to visits, to call periodically during the few first weeks after discharge to determine whether the patient is improving. These contacts will help the patient to feel valued and connected to others. Lack of continuity is thought to contribute to significant suicide mortality after hospital discharge (Hulten and Wasserman 1998)' (Murray and Hauenstein 2008, p.916).

Appropriate referrals to professionals in the community, and available resources and support are important. The community nurse/therapist requires adequate information to continue with effective interventions following discharge. In addition, engaging family and friends in the patient's ongoing care and finding sources of help in the community, such as church groups, clubhouses, drop-in centres or other social groups, is a necessary task.

Case study 2 in Box 6.8 gives an example of how ADPIE can be applied in practice.

Box 6.8   Case study: Julie.

Situation

Julie is a 19 year old girl with an intellectual disability. Julie lives in a group home and sees her family twice a year. She is being admitted for her fifth suicide attempt. Julie has been cutting and threatening suicide for a number of years and is well known to the staff on the unit where you work. The staff appear to be somewhat hostile toward Julie and view her cutting and suicide attempts as attention-seeking behaviour. They do not feel Julie should be admitted and they believe this self-injurious behaviour should be ignored. Julie's care is assigned to you during this evening shift.

Nurse's interpretation

The nurse recognises that Julie's behaviour indicates that she is probably struggling with a number of stressors and intolerable loss. She also recognises that Julie is vulnerable due to her intellectual disability. The nurse notices that Julie appears to feel helpless, hopeless and powerless to change her situation. The nurse also recognises that ignoring this suicidal behaviour will probably escalate the behaviour. Although the nurse recognises that it may not be uncommon for the staff to react this way she also realises that this attitude may impact on the care that Julie receives.

Nurse's action

The nurse establishes a therapeutic relationship with Julie and performs a comprehensive assessment of risk, being very careful to be calm and patient and to listen to Julie's story. The nurse also asks curious questions to understand if Julie has been harmed in any way due to her vulnerability and what Julie perceives her stressors to be. The nurse is non-judgmental and treats Julie with positive regard. Interventions are planned according to the assessment of risk and information gathering. The nurse also approaches the nurse manager to discuss Julie's case and the staff's reaction and suggests that an interprofessional case conference be planned to assist Julie to deal with issues in her life and at her group home. The nurse also suggests a possible in-service regarding repetitive suicidal behaviour.

Legal considerations in caring for people at risk to self

Mental health nurses must understand patients' legal rights and be able to explain them clearly (Murray and Hauenstein 2008). Patients have the right to self-determination. They also have the right to privacy and anonymity unless disclosure is needed to provide safety. Patients also have the right of beneficence, which is the right to be free from harm. Physically restraining or hospitalising patients against their will has the potential for both physical and emotional harm and should be used only under the threat of imminent suicide or psychosis (Murray and Hauenstein 2008).

Confidentiality

The concept of confidentiality is described as the safeguarding of information acquired within a professional relationship, except when doing so would cause significant harm (Canadian Nurses Association (CNA) 2002). The mental health nurse needs to be very clear and specific when explaining the limits of confidentiality to the patient. Protecting the patient's right to confidentiality is of particular concern when dealing with a minor child. The nurse must always consider informing the child's parents or legal guardians if he/she has concerns regarding self-harm or suicidal behaviour (RNAO 2008).

Documentation

Although documentation is a standard of nursing practice and is an integral part of the assessment and care of clients at risk of suicidal ideation there is no consensus on a standard way to document suicide risk assessments. It is important for each organisation to develop policies that guide systematic, accurate and thorough documentation.

Competence

The competent patient can reason and make decisions based on sound interpretations of the information available. A patient may be deemed incompetent when his or her judgment is impaired (e.g. psychosis, influence of drugs or alcohol). The nurse must assess the patient's competence on an ongoing basis, especially as it is related to informed consent and a no self-harm contract.

No self-harm contract

'The nurse should consider a no self-harm contract only after a thorough assessment of the patient (Simon 1999). The nurse must consider several factors in

making a no self-harm contract with a patient. The patient must be competent to enter into such a contract. Patients under the influence of drugs or alcohol or experiencing psychoses are not competent to make no self-harm contracts' (Murray and Hauenstein 2008, p.912).

It is important that the no self-harm contract be considered as *the patient's commitment to keep him- or herself safe* rather than *a promise to the nurse not to harm him-/herself*. A safety plan should also be discussed with the patient to deal with suicidal ideation in order to avert the progression to suicidal behaviour.

Involuntary/voluntary admission

Voluntary admission is ideal and protects the rights of the patient; however, involuntary admission to hospital is necessary when the patient's safety or someone else's safety cannot be ensured. Different jurisdictions may have differing criteria for involuntary admission and it is important for the mental health nurse to be aware of the criteria for determination.

Survivors of suicide and trauma

'In the suicide prevention field, "survivor" is a word used to describe someone who has lost a significant other to suicide. It does not refer to those who have made a suicide attempt and survived' (Ball and White 2005, p.4).

'Worldwide, about 1 million persons die of suicide each year (World Health Organization 2004). Each suicide has an impact on an average of 6–7 survivors, so that 6 million persons lose someone close to them due to suicide each year (Tondo and Baldessarini 2001). Suicide has devastating effects on everyone it touches, especially family and close friends. Undue and prolonged suffering can be caused by the sudden shock, the unanswered questions of "why," and potentially the discovery of the body (Knieper 1999). Suicide bereavement is different than that experienced by families whose loved one's death is not self-inflicted. The grieving over the way the death occurred, the social processes affecting the survivor and the effect of the suicide on the family converge to establish a grieving process that is unique (Jordan 2001)' (Murray and Hauenstein 2008, p.907).

It is important for the healthcare professional to be aware of available postvention services.

Postvention includes Critical Incident Stress Debriefing (CISD) for victims and survivors of the event and Critical Incident Stress Management (CISM) for organisations to provide services to employed professionals and emergency service personnel.

CISD

The primary goals of debriefing are to accelerate recovery processes in people who are experiencing stress reactions to abnormal traumatic events and to mitigate the impact of the critical incident on those who were victims of the event, be they primary victims, i.e. those directly traumatised by the event; secondary victims, such as emergency services personnel who witnessed or managed the traumatic event; or tertiary victims, i.e. family, friends and those to whom the traumatic event may be indirectly communicated to. The secondary objectives include:

- prevention or mitigation of post traumatic stress disorder (PTSD);
- reassurance that the stress response is normal and controllable and recovery is likely;
- education about the stress response;
- emotional ventilation;
- screening for people who need additional assessment or therapy;
- referral to appropriate services.

CISM

CISM is a multidimensional stress management service for healthcare professionals and their families. The programme should include education and prevention programmes, CISD, a resource and referral network and family education and support programmes. The programme needs to be flexible enough to provide individualised support when necessary due to the varying stress responses of different professionals.

The stress response can be either acute or delayed. It may be an immediate reaction to a specific incident or it may be a delayed response to unsuccessful attempts to cope with a critical incident(s) (Figley 1995). The individual reaction of the mental health nurse can depend on several factors, such as the intensity and duration of the exposure, and the nurse's interpretation of having been at risk. Also the individual's attitude towards his or her perception of training and preparedness, job satisfaction and rescue efforts, as well as personal attributes and successes or failures with coping, and the resources available can influence the individual nurse's response. Nurses need to recognise and deal effectively with the stressors inherent in their profession. However, the need to seek mental health support is often seen as a sign of weakness. There is a stigma associated with seeking out professional support as this may raise questions related to their ability to continue in their work. There is a cost to caring (Murray and Hauenstein 2008, p.916). When we listen to clients' stories of fear, pain and suffering, we may feel similar pain and suffering because we care.

To care successfully for suicidal patients or others prone to crises, the nurse must engage in an active programme of self-care. Such a programme begins with proper rest, exercise and nutrition so that the nurse can better manage stress physiologically. Self-monitoring of symptoms is the next step. Nurses should also be alert to symptoms of PTSD. Caring for suicidal patients is highly stressful and may lead to compassion fatigue (Figley 1995). The nurse who experiences compassion fatigue may begin to have symptoms that reflect the early stage of PTSD. It is important for nurses to develop cognitive coping skills, to seek help when needed and to engage in stress reduction exercises. Those who have an enormous capacity for feeling and expressing empathy tend to be more at risk of compassion fatigue. The most effective caregivers are often the most vulnerable for this reason.

Conclusion

Risk to self includes suicidal behaviour (varying degrees of self-harm, including self-injurious behaviour and self-mutilation), self neglect (both physical and social) and vulnerability (being at risk of harm from others). Risk to self behaviour must be understood in the context of biological, psychological and social theories and the determinants of health. It is important for the mental health nurse to recognise risk and protective factors for risk to self and invitations to help, in order to understand the behaviour from the patient's perspective. It is important for interventions to be based on a comprehensive assessment of risk. Suicidal behaviour is often a means of communication that life has become difficult and intolerable, and there is a feeling of powerlessness, helplessness and hopelessness that life circumstances will not change. Establishment of a therapeutic relationship with the patient is essential to foster hope and the expectation of recovery. There is a cost to caring and nurses must participate in self-care and postvention both personally and professionally.

Acknowledgements

The chapter authors would like to thank the following for their kind permission to reproduce some of the text and tables contained within this chapter that originally appeared in the following sources: Ramsay *et al.* (2004), Murray and Hauenstein (2008), and the Registered Nurses' Association of Ontario (2008).

References

Abrams, R.C., Lachs, M., McAvay, G., Keohane, D.J. & Bruce, M.L. (2002) Predictors of self-neglect in community-dwelling elders. *American Journal of Psychiatry*, **159**, 1724–1730.

Adam, K.S., Keler, A., West, M., Larose, S. & Goszer, L.B. (1994) Parental representation in suicidal adolescents: a controlled study. *Australian and New Zealand Journal of Psychiatry*, **28**, 418–425.

Adler, G. & Buie, D.H. Jr (1996) Aloneness and borderline psychopathology: possible relevance of child development issues. In: *Essential Papers on Suicide* (eds J.T. Maltsberger & M.J. Goldblatt), pp. 356–378. New York University Press, New York.

Ahrens, B., Linden, M., Zaske, H. & Berzewski, H. (2000) Suicidal behavior – symptom or disorder? *Comprehensive Psychiatry*, **41**, 116–121.

Alexopoulos, G.S., Bruce, M.L., Hull, J., Sireej, J.A. & Kakumo, T. (1999) Clinical determinant of suicidal ideation and behaviour in geriatric depression. *Archives of General Psychiatry*, **56**, 1048–1053.

American Psychiatric Association (APA) (2003) *Practice Guideline for the Assessment and Treatment of Patients with Suicidal Behaviors.* APA, Arlington.

Anderson, M. (1999) Waiting for harm: deliberate self-harm and suicide in young people – a review of the literature. *Journal of Psychiatric and Mental Health Nursing*, **6**, 91–100.

Angst, J., Angst, F. & Stassen, H.S. (1999) Suicide risk in patients with major depressive disorder. *Journal of Clinical Psychiatry*, **6**, 57–62.

Aoun, S. (1999) Deliberate self-harm in rural Western Australia: results of an intervention study. *Australian and New Zealand Journal of Mental and Health Nursing*, **8**, 65–73.

Appleby, L., Shaw, J., Amos, T., *et al.* (1999a) Suicide within 12 months of contact with mental health services: national clinical survey. *British Medical Journal*, **318**, 1235–1239.

Appleby, L., Cooper, J., Amos, T. & Faragher, B. (1999b) Psychological autopsy study of suicides by people aged under 35. *British Journal of Psychiatry*, **175**, 168–174.

Armitage, C.J. (2005) Can the theory of planned behavior predict the maintenance of physical activity? *Health Psychology*, **24**, 235–245.

Baldessarini, R.J. & Hennen, J. (2004) Genetics of suicide: an overview. *Harvard Review of Psychiatry*, **12**, 1–13.

Baldessarini, R.J., Tondo, L. & Hennen, J. (1999) Effects of lithium treatment and its discontinuation on suicidal behavior in bipolar manic-depressive disorders. *Journal of Clinical Psychiatry*, **60**, 77–84.

Ball, B. & White, J. (2005) Wondering and wanderings: ongoing conversations about suicide prevention. *Visions: BC's Mental Health and Addictions Journal*, **2**, 4–5.

Barrett, F.M., King, A., Levy, J., Maticka-Tyndale, E. & McKay, A. (1997) Sexuality in Canada. In: *The International Encyclopedia of Sexuality, Vol. 1* (ed. R. Francoeur), pp. 221–343. Continuum Publishing, New York.

Beck, A.T. (2002) *Cognitive therapy of borderline personality disorder and attempted suicide.* Paper presented at the conference of the Treatment and Research Advancements Association for Personality Disorders, Bethesda, Maryland.

Beck, A.T. & Emery, G. (1985) *Anxiety Disorders and Phobias: A Cognitive Perspective.* Basic Books, New York.

Beck, A.T., Ward, C.H., Mendelson, M., Mock, J. & Erbaugh, J. (1961) An inventory for measuring depression. *Archives of General Psychiatry*, **4**, 561–571.

Beck, A.T., Kovacs, M. & Weissman, A. (1979a) Assessment of suicidal intention: the scale for suicidal ideation. *Journal of Consulting and Clinical Psychology*, **47**, 343–352.

Beck, A.T., Rush, A.J., Shaw, B.F. & Emery, G. (1979b) *Cognitive Therapy in Depression.* Guilford Press, New York.

Beck, A.T., Steer, R.A., Kovacs, M. & Garrison, B. (1985) Hopelessness and eventual suicide: a 10 year prospective study of patients hospitalized with suicide ideation. *American Journal of Psychology*, **142**, 559–563.

Beck, A.T., Brown, G.K. & Steer, R.A. (1997) Psychometric characteristics of the Scale for Suicide Ideation with psychiatric outpatients. *Behaviour Research and Therapy*, **35**, 1039–1046.

Berg, I.K. (1994) *Family-Based Services: A Solution-Focused Approach.* W.W. Norton, New York.

Berglund, M. & Ojehagen, A. (1998) The influence of alcohol drinking and alcohol use disorders on psychiatric disorders and suicidal behaviour. *Alcoholism: Clinical and Experimental Research*, **22**, 3335–3455.

Berman, A.L. (1988) Fictional depiction of suicide in television films and imitation effects. *American Journal of Psychiatry*, **145**, 982–986.

Blumenthal, S.J. & Kupfer, D.J. (1990) *Suicide Over the Life Cycle: Risk Factors, Assessment and Treatment of Suicidal Patients.* American Psychiatric Press, Washington, DC.

Bodfish, J.W. (1999) *Clinical conditions associated with self-injury: using comorbidity patterns to guide the search for mechanisms and treatments.* Paper presented at NICHD Conference on SLB, 6–7 December, Rockville, Maryland.

Borthwick-Duffy, S.A. (1994) Prevalence of destructive behaviors: a study of aggression, self-injury and property destruction. In: *Destructive Behaviors in Developmental Disabilities* (eds T. Thompson & D.B. Gray). Sage, London.

Bostwick, J.M. & Pankratz, V.S. (2000) Affective disorders and suicide risk: a reexamination. *American Journal of Psychiatry*, **157**, 1925–1932.

Brieger, P., Ehrt, U., Bloeink, R. & Marneros, A. (2002) Consequences of comorbid personality disorders in major depression. *Journal of Nervous and Mental Disease*, **190**, 304–309.

Brock, A., Baker, A., Griffiths, C., Jackson, G., Fegan, G. & Marshall, D. (2006) Suicide trends and geographical variations in the United Kingdom, 1991–2004. *Health Statistics Quarterly*, **31**, 6–22.

Canadian Nurses Association (CNA) (2002) *Code of Ethics*. Canadian Nurses Association, Ottawa.

Cantor, C.H. & Baume, P.J. (1998) Access to methods of suicide: what impact? *Australian and New Zealand Journal of Psychiatry*, **32**, 8–14.

Catallozzi, M., Pletcher, J.R. & Schwarz, D.F. (2001) Prevention of suicide in adolescents. *Current Opinion in Pediatrics*, **13**, 417–422.

Center for Disease Control and Prevention (CDC) (2005) *Suicide: Facts at a Glance*. Available at http://www.cdc.gov/ncipc/dvp/suicide/SuicideDataSheet.pdf (accessed 3 March 2008).

Cerel, J., Fristad, M.A., Weller, E.B. & Weller, R.A. (1999) Suicide-bereaved children and adolescents: a controlled longitudinal examination. *Journal of the American Academy of Child and Adolescent Psychiatry*, **38**, 672–679.

Clark, D.C. & Goebel-Fabbri, A.E. (1998) Lifetime risk of suicide in major affective disorders. In: *Harvard Medical School Guide to Assessment and Intervention in Suicide* (ed. D. Jacobs), pp. 270–286. Jossey-Bass, San Francisco.

Conwell, Y. & Henderson, R.E. (1996) Neuropsychiatry of suicide. In: *Neuropsychiatry* (eds B.S. Fogel, R.B. Schiffer & S.M. Rao). Williams & Wilkins, Baltimore.

Conwell, Y., Duberstein, P.R., Cox, C., Herrmann, J., Forbes, N. & Caine, E.D. (1998) Age differences in behaviors leading to completed suicide. *American Journal of Geriatric Psychiatry*, **6**, 122–126.

Corcoran, J. (1998) Solution-focused practice with middle and high school at-risk youths. *Social Work in Education*, **20**, 232–242.

Corsini, R.J. & Wedding, D. (2005) *Current Psychotherapies*, 7th edn. Brooks/Cole, Monterey.

Cutcliffe, J.R. (2003) *From 'Policing' to Reconnecting: The Problem of Suicide in Canada*. BC Partners for Mental Health and Addictions Information. Available at http://www.heretohelp.bc.ca/publications/suicide/bck/web/1 (accessed 17 April 2008).

deGraaf, T.K. (1998) A family therapeutic approach to transgenerational traumatization. *Family Processes*, **37**, 233–242.

DeShazer, S. (1988) *Clues: Investigating Solutions in Brief Therapy*. Norton, New York.

DeWilde, E.J., Kienhorst, I.C.W.M., Diekstra, R.F.W. & Wolters, W.H.G. (1992) The relationship between adolescent suicide attempts and life events in childhood and adolescence. *American Journal of Psychiatry*, **149**, 45–51.

Eggert, L.L. & Thompson, E.A. (2002) Preliminary effects of brief school-based prevention approaches for reducing youth suicide: risk behaviours, depression and drug involvement. *Journal of Child and Adolescent Psychiatric Nursing*, **15**, 48–64.

Eng, P.M., Rimm, E.B., Fitzmaurice, G. & Kawachi, I. (2002) Social ties and change in social ties in relation to subsequent total and cause-specific mortality and coronary heart disease incidence in men. *American Journal of Epidemiology*, **155**, 700–709.

Fairbairn, G. (1995) *Contemplating Suicide: The Language and Ethics of Self-harm.* Routledge, London.

Favaro, A. & Santonastaso, P. (2000) Self-injurious behavior nervosa. *Journal of Nervous and Mental Disease*, **188**, 537–542.

Fergusson, D.M., Woodward, L.J. & Horwood, L.J. (2000) Risk factors and life processes associated with the onset of suicidal behaviour during adolescence and early adulthood. *Psychological Medicine*, **30**, 23–39.

Ferreira de Castro, E., Cunha, M.A., Pimenta, F. & Costa, I. (1998) Parasuicide and mental disorders. *Acta Psychiatrica Scandinavica*, **97**, 25–31.

Figley, C. (1995) *Compassion Fatigue.* Brunnwe/Mazel, New York.

Foster, T., Gillespie, K., McClelland, R. & Patterson, C. (1999) Risk factors for suicide independent of *DSM-III-R* axis I disorder: case-control psychological autopsy study in Northern Ireland. *British Journal of Psychiatry*, **175**, 175–179.

Friedman, R.A. (2006) Violence and mental illness: how strong is the link? *New England Journal of Medicine*, **20**, 2064–2066.

Gates, B. (2000) Self-injurious behaviour: reviewing evidence for best practice. *British Journal of Nursing*, **9**, 96–102.

Ge, X., Conger, R.D. & Elder, G.H. Jr (1996) Coming of age too early: pubertal influences on girls' vulnerability to psychological distress. *Child Development*, **67**, 3386–3400.

Gibson, P. (1994) Gay male and lesbian youth suicide. In: *Report of the Secretary's Task Force on Youth Suicide* (ed. M. Feinleif), pp. 131–142. Department of Health and Human Services, Washington, DC.

Glowinski, A.L., Bucholz, K.K., Nelson, E.C., *et al.* (2001) Suicide attempts in an adolescent female twin sample. *Journal of the American Academy of Child and Adolescent Psychiatry*, **40**, 1300–1307.

Goldney, R.D. (1985) Parental representation in young women who attempt suicide. *Acta Psychiatry Scandinavia*, **72**, 230–232.

Goldney, R.D. (1989) Suicide: role of the media. *Australian and New Zealand Journal of Psychiatry*, **23**, 30–34.

Gould, M.S. & Kramer, R.A. (2001) Youth suicide prevention. *Suicide and Life Threatening Behaviour*, **31**, 6–31.

Gould, M.S., Fisher, P., Parides, M., Flory, M. & Shaffer, D. (1996) Psychosocial risk factors of child and adolescent completed suicide. *Archives of General Psychiatry*, **53**, 1155–1162.

Grant, B.F. & Hasin, D.S. (1999) Suicidal ideation among the United States drinking population: results from the National Longitudinal Alcohol Epidemiologic Survey. *Journal of Studies on Alcohol*, **60**, 422–429.

Gunnell, D. & Middelton, N. (2003) National suicide rates as an indicator of the effect of suicide on premature mortality. *The Lancet*, **362**, 961–962.

Halliday, S. & Mackrell, K. (1998) Psychological interventions in self-injurious behavior. *British Journal of Psychiatry*, **172**, 395–400.

Hawton, K. (2000) Sex and suicide: gender differences in suicidal behaviour. *British Journal of Psychiatry*, **177**, 484–485.

Hawton, K., Fagg, J., Simkin, S., Bale, E. & Bond, A. (1997) Trends in deliberate self-harm in Oxford, 1985–1995. *British Journal of Psychiatry*, **171**, 556–560.

Health Canada (1994) *Suicide in Canada: Update of the Report of the Task Force on Suicide in Canada*. Health Canada, Ottawa.

Health Canada (2002) A *Report on Mental Illnesses in Canada*. Available at http://www.phac-aspc.gc.ca/publicat/miic-mmac/ (accessed 20 January 2008).

Hegadoren, K. & McCabe, S. (2008) Psychopharmacology. In: *Psychiatric Nursing for Canadian Practice* (eds W. Austin & M.A. Boyd), pp. 196–241. Lippincott Williams and Wilkins, Philadelphia.

Hendin, H. (1991) Psychodynamics of suicide, with particular reference to the young. *American Journal of Psychiatry*, **148**, 1150–1158.

Hogg, M.A. & Abrams, D. (1988) *Social Identifications: A Social Psychology of Intergroup Relations and Group Processes*. Routledge, London.

Holkup, P.A. (2003) Evidence-based protocol: elderly suicide-secondary prevention *Journal of Gerontological Nursing*, **29**, 6–17.

Hulten, A. & Wasserman, D. (1998) Lack of continuity: a problem in the care of young suicides. *Acta Psychiatrica Scandinavica*, **97**, 326–333.

Hwalek, M.A. (1996) The association of elder abuse and substance abuse in the Illinois elder abuse system. *The Gerontologist*, **36**(5), 694–700.

Isometsa, E.T. & Lonnqvist, J.K. (1998) Suicide attempts preceding completed suicide. *British Journal of Psychiatry*, **173**, 531–535.

Jamison, K.R. (1999) *Night Falls Fast: Understanding Suicide*. Knopf, New York.

Jobes, D. (2000) Collaborating to prevent suicide: a clinical research perspective. *Suicide and Life Threatening Behaviour*, **30**, 164–173.

Jobes, D.A., Berman, A.L., O'Carroll, P.W., Eastgard, S. & Knickmeyer, S. (1996) The Kurt Cobain suicide crisis: perspectives from research, public health, and the news media. *Suicide and Life-Threatening Behavior*, **26**(3), 260–271.

Johnson, I. & Sigler, R. (2000) Forced sexual intercourse among intimates. *Journal of Interpersonal Violence*, **15**(1), 95–108.

Johnson, J. & Adams, J. (1996) Self-neglect in later life. *Health and Social Care in the Community*, **4**, 26–33.

Jordan, J.R. (2001) Is suicide bereavement different? A reassessment of the literature. *Suicide and Life Threatening Behaviour*, **31**, 91–102.

Kapur, N. (2005) Management of self-harm in adults: which way now? *British Journal of Psychiatry*, **187**, 497–499.

Kapur, N., House, A., Creed, F., Feldman, E., Friedman, T. & Guthrie, E. (1998) Management of deliberate self-poisoning in four teaching hospitals: descriptive study. *British Medical Journal*, **316**, 831–832.

Kienhorst, I.W.M., De Wilde, E.J. & Diekstra, R.F.W. (1995) Suicidal behaviour in adolescents. *Archives of Suicide Research*, **1**, 185–209.

Klimes-Dougan, B., Free, K., Ronsaville, D., Stilwell, J., Welsh, C.J. & Radke-Yarrow, M. (1999) Suicidal ideation and attempts: a longitudinal investigation of children of depressed and well mothers. *Journal of the American Academy of Child and Adolescent Psychiatry*, **38**(6), 651–659.

Knieper, A.J. (1999) The suicide survivor's grief and recovery. *Suicide and Life Threatening Behaviour*, **29**, 353–364.

Kohlmeier, R.E., McMahan, C.A. & DiMaio, V.J.M. (2001) Suicide by firearms: a fifteen year experience. *American Journal of Forensic Medicine and Pathology*, **22**, 337–340.

Kushner, H.I. & Sterk, C.I. (2005) The limits of social capital: Durkheim, suicide, and social cohesion. *American Journal of Public Health*, **95**, 1139–1143.

Lachs, M., Williams, C., O'Brien, S., Hurst, L. & Horwitz, R. (1996) Older adults: an 11-year longitudinal study of adult protective service use. *Archives of International Medicine*, **156**, 449–453.

Lauder, W. (1998) Constructs of self-neglect: a multiple case study design. *Nursing Inquiry*, **6**, 48–57.

Lawlink, N.S.W. (2003) *Sexual Abuse of People with Disability*. Available at http://www.lawlink.nsw.gov.au/cpd.nsf/pages/blyth (accessed 20 May 2005).

Leenaars, A.A. (1998) *Suicide Notes: Predictive Clues and Patterns*. Human Sciences Press, New York.

Leenaars, A.A. (2004) *Psychotherapy with Suicidal People: A Person-Centered Approach*. John Wiley & Sons, Toronto. Available at http://www.aeschiconference.unibe.ch/Psychoth_with_Suicidal%20People.html (accessed 23 April 2008).

Lester, D. (2000) Alcoholism, substance abuse, and suicide. In: *Comprehensive Textbook of Suicidology* (eds R.W. Maris, A. Berman & M.M. Silverman), pp. 357–375. Guilford Press, New York.

Levenkron, S. (1998) *Cutting: Understanding and Overcoming Self-Mutilation*. Norton, London.

Lewis, M.H. & Bodfish, J.W. (1998) Repetitive behaviour in autism. *Mental Retardation and Developmental Disability Research Reviews*, **4**, 80–89.

Link, B.G., Phelan, J.C., Bresnahan, M., Stueve, A. & Pescosolido, B. (1999) Public conceptions of mental illness: labels, causes, dangerousness, and social distance. *American Journal of Public Health*, **89**, 1328–1333.

Lopez, F.G. & Brennan, K.A. (2000) Dynamic processes underlying adult attachment organization: toward an attachment theoretical perspective on the health and effective self. *Journal of Counseling Psychology*, **47**, 283–300.

MacDonald, M. (1994) Sexuality and the criminal law in Canada: issues for sex educators and therapists. *Canadian Journal of Sexuality*, **3**, 15–23.

Machoian, L. (2001) Cutting voices: self-injury in three adolescent girls. *Journal of Psychosocial Nursing and Mental Health Services*, **39**, 22–29.

MacMillan, H.L., Fleming, J.E., Streiner, D.L., *et al.* (2001) Childhood abuse and lifetime psychopathology in a community sample. *American Journal of Psychiatry*, **158**(11), 1878–1883.

Maine, S., Shute, R. & Martin, G. (2001) Educating parents about youth suicide: knowledge, response to suicidal statements, attitudes, and intention to help. *Suicide and Life-Threatening Behaviour*, **31**, 320–332.

Mann, J.J., Brent, D.A. & Arango, V. (2001) The neurobiology and genetics of suicide and attempted suicide: a focus on the serotonergic system. *Neuropsychopharmacology*, **24**, 467–477.

Marriage and Family Encyclopedia (2008) *Suicide: The Epidemiology of Suicide, Theories of Suicide, Marital Status and the Family, the Protective Effect of Children*. Available at http://family.jrank.org/pages/1658/Suicide-Theories-Suicide.html (accessed 13 March 2008).

McAllister, M. (2003) Multiple meanings of self harm: a critical review. *International Journal of Mental Health Nursing*, **12**, 177–185.

McGoldrick, M. (1992) The legacy of loss. In: *Living Beyond Loss: Death in the Family* (eds F. Walsh & M. McGoldrick), pp.104–129. Norton, New York.

McKeown, R.E., Garrison, C.Z., Cuffe, S.P., Waller, J.L., Jackson, K.L. & Addy, C.L. (1998) Incidence and predictors of suicidal behaviours in a longitudinal sample of young adolescents. *Journal of the American Academy of Child and Adolescent Psychiatry*, **37**, 612–619.

Meyer, J.H., McMain, S., Kennedy, S.H., *et al.* (2003) Dysfunctional attitudes and 5-HT$_2$ receptors during depression and self-harm. *American Journal of Psychiatry*, **160**, 90–99.

Minino, A.M., Heron, M.P., Arias, E., Murphy, S.L. & Kochanek, K.D. (2007) Deaths: final data for 2000. *National Vital Statistics Reports*, **55**(19), 1–120. Available at http://www.cdc.gov/nchs/data/nvsr/nvsr55/nvsr55_19.pdf (accessed 3 May 2008).

Minuchin, S. & Fishman, C. (1981) *Family Therapy Techniques*. Harvard University Press, Cambridge, Massachusetts.

Morrison, L.L. & L'Heureux, J. (2001) Suicide and gay/lesbian/bisexual youth: implications for clinicians. *Journal of Adolescence*, **24**, 39–49.

Mosciki, E.K. (1998) Epidemiology of suicide. In: *Harvard Medical School Guide to Assessment and Intervention in Suicide* (ed. D. Jacobs), pp. 40–51. Jossey-Bass, San Francisco.

Murray, B.L. (2003) Self-harm among adolescents with developmental disabilities: what are they trying to tell us? *Psychosocial Nursing and Mental Health Services*, 41, 36–45.

Murray, B.L. & Hauenstein, E.J. (2008) Self harm and suicidal behaviour: children, adolescents, and adults. In: *Psychiatric Nursing for Canadian Practice* (eds W. Austin & M.A. Boyd), pp. 898–922. Lippincott Williams & Wilkins, Philadelphia.

Murray, B.L. & Wright, K. (2006) Integration of a suicide risk assessment and intervention approach: the perspective of youth. *Journal of Psychiatric Mental Health Nursing*, **13**, 157–164.

NANYouth (2004) *Aboriginal Suicide Statistics*. Available at http://www.nandecade.ca/article/71.asp (accessed 10 August 2005).

National Institute of Mental Health (2005) *Glossary*. Available at http://science.education.nih.gov/supplements/nih5/mental/other/glossary.htm (accessed 13 March 2008).

Neeleman, J. (1998) Regional suicide rates in The Netherlands: does religion still play a role? *International Journal of Epidemiology*, **27**, 466–472.

Nemeroff, C.B., Compton, M.T. & Berger, J. (2001) The depressed suicidal patient: assessment and treatment. *Annals of American Academy of Sciences*, **932**, 1–23.

New Zealand Guidelines Group (NZGG) (2003) *The Assessment and Management of People at Risk of Suicide*. NZGG, Wellington.

North American Nursing Diagnosis Association International (NANDA) (2006) *Nursing Diagnoses: Definition and Classification, 2005–2006*. NANDA, Philadelphia.

O'Connor, R.C., Armitage, C.J. & Lorna Gray, L. (2006) The role of clinical and social cognitive variables. *British Journal of Clinical Psychology*, **45**, 465–481.

O'Hanlon, W.H. & Werner-Davis, M. (1989) *In Search of Solutions: A New Direction in Psychotherapy*. Norton, New York.

O'Loughlin, S. & Sherwood, J. (2005) A 20-year review of deliberate self-harm in a British Town: 1981–2000. *Social Psychiatry and Social Epidemiology*, **40**, 446–453.

Oliver, C. (1995) Self-injurious behaviour in children with learning disabilities: recent advances in assessment and intervention. *Journal of Child Psychology*, **30**, 909–927.

Oliver, C., Murphy, G.H. & Corbett, J.A. (1987) Self-injurious behaviour in people with mental handicap: a total population study. *Journal of Mental Deficiency Research*, **31**, 147–162.

Owens, D., Horrocks, J. & House, A. (2002) Fatal and non-fatal repetition of self-harm. Systematic review. *British Journal of Psychiatry*, **181**, 193–199.

Parris, T. (2006) *On Suicide.* Available at http://www.Parris.com/psychology/abnormal/suicide/section1.html (accessed 18 April 2008).

Phillips, D.P. & Carstensen, L.L. (1986) Clustering of teenage suicides after television news stories. *New England Journal of Medicine,* **315,** 685–689.

Platt, S. (1993) The social transmission of parasuicide: is there a modeling effect? *Crisis,* **14,** 23–31.

Plomin, R., Owen, M.J. & McGuffin, P. (1994) The genetic basis of complex human behaviours. *Science,* **264,** 1733–1739.

Poijula, S., Wahlberg, K.E. & Dyregrov, A. (2001) Adolescent suicide and suicide contagion in three secondary schools. *Journal of Emergency Mental Health,* **3,** 163–168.

Preuss, U.W., Schuckit, M.A., Smith, T.L., *et al.* (2002) Comparison of 3190 alcohol-dependent individuals with and without suicide attempts. *Alcoholism: Clinical and Experimental Research,* **26,** 471–477.

Prigerson, H.G. & Slimack, M.J. (1999) Gender differences in clinical correlates of suicidality among young adults. *Journal of Nervous and Mental Disease,* **187,** 23–31.

Public Health Agency of Canada (2000) *Leading Causes of Death and Hospitalization in Canada.* Available at http://www.phac-aspc.gc.ca/publicat/lcd-pcd97/index.html (accessed 15 August 2005).

Qin, P., Agergbo, E. & Mortensen, P.B. (2003) Suicide risk in relationship to socioeconomic, demographic, psychiatric, and familial factors: a national register-based study of all suicides in Denmark, 1981–1997. *American Journal of Psychiatry,* **160,** 765–772.

Radloff, L. (1977) The CES-D scale: a self-report depression scale for research in the general population. *Applied Psychological Measurement,* **1,** 385–401.

Radomsky, E.D., Haas, G.L., Mann, J.J. & Sweeney, J.A. (1999) Suicidal behaviour in patients with schizophrenia and other psychotic disorders. *American Journal Psychiatry,* **156,** 1590–1595.

Ramsay, R.F., Yanney, B.L., Lang, W.A. & Kinzel, T. (2004) *Suicide Intervention Handbook.* Living Works Education, Calgary.

Ramsay, R.F., Tanny, B.L., Taierney, R.J. & Lang, W.A. (1994) *Suicide Intervention Handbook.* Living Works Education, Calgary.

Rathbone-McCuan, E. & Bricker-Jenkins, M. (1992) A general framework for elder self-neglect. In: *Self-Neglecting Elders: A Clinical Dilemma* (eds E. Rathbone-McCuan & D.R. Fabian), pp. 13–24. Auburn House, New York.

Registered Nurses' Association of Ontario (RNAO) (2006) *Establishing Therapeutic Relationships* (Revised). RNAO, Toronto.

Registered Nurses' Association of Ontario (2008) *Assessment and Care of Adults at Risk for Suicidal Ideation and Behaviour.* RNAO, Toronto.

Reinherz, H.Z., Giaconia, R.M., Silverman, A.B., *et al.* (1995) Early psychosocial risks for adolescent suicidal ideation and attempts. *Journal of the American Academy of Child and Adolescent Psychiatry,* **34,** 599–611.

Remafedi, G., Farrow, J. & Deisher, R. (1991) Risk factors for attempted suicide in gay and bisexual youth. *Pediatrics*, **87**, 869–875.

Rew, L., Thomas, N., Horner, S. Resnick, M. & Beuhring, T. (2001) Correlates of recent suicide attempts in a tri-ethnic group of adolescents. *Journal of Nursing Scholarship*, **4**, 361–367.

Rioch, S. (1995) *Suicidal Children & Adolescence: Crisis and Preventative Care.* Celia Publications, Durham.

Robertson, M.M., Trimble, M.R. & Lees, A.J. (1989) Self-injurious behaviour and the Gilles de la Tourette syndrome: a clinical study and review of the literature. *Psychological Medicine*, **19**, 611–625.

Rogers, C. (1980) *A Way of Being.* Houghton Mifflin, Boston.

Rosenberg, N.K. (1993) Psychotherapy of the suicidal patient. *Acta Psychiatrica Scandinavica*, **371**, 54–56.

Rotheram-Borus, M.J. & Fernandez, M.I. (1995) Sexual orientation and developmental challenges experienced by gay and lesbian youths. *Suicide and Life Threatening Behaviour*, **23**, 26–34.

Roy, A. (1989) Suicide. In: *Comprehensive Textbook of Psychiatry* (eds H.I. Kaplan & B.J. Sadock), pp. 1414–1427. Williams & Wilkins, Baltimore.

Russell, S.T. & Joyner, K. (2001) Adolescent sexual orientation and suicide risk: evidence from a nation study. *American Journal of Public Health*, **9**(8), 1276–1281.

Savin-Williams, R. (1990) *Gay and Lesbian Youth: Expressions of Identity.* Hemisphere, New York.

Schmidtke, A. & Hafner, H. (1988) The Werther effect after television films: new evidence for an old hypothesis. *Psychological Medicine*, **18**, 665–676.

Schroeder, S., Oster-Granite, M., Berkson, G., *et al.* (2001) Self-injurious behaviour: gene–brain–behaviour relationships. *Mental Retardation and Developmental Disabilities*, **7**, 3–12.

Schulsinger, F., Kety, S.S., Rosenthal, D. & Wender, P.H. (1979) A family study of suicide. In: *Origins, Prevention, and Treatment of Affective Disorders* (eds M. Schou & E. Stromgren), pp. 277–287. Academic, New York.

Sheeran, P., Orbell, S. & Trafimow, D. (1999) Does the temporal stability of behavioral intentions moderate intention–behavior and past behavior–future behavior relations? *Personality and Social Psychology Bulletin*, **25**, 721–730.

Shoumitro, D. (1996) Self-injurious behaviour as part of genetic syndromes. *British Journal of Psychiatry*, **172**, 385–388.

Silove, D., George, G. & Bhavani-Sankaram, V. (1987) Parasuicide: interaction between inadequate parenting and recent interpersonal stress. *Australian and New Zealand Journal of Psychiatry*, **21**, 221–228.

Simon, R.I. (1999) The suicide prevention contract: clinical, legal and risk management issues. *Journal of the American Academy of Psychiatry and the Law*, **27**, 445–450.

Sinason, V. (1992) *Mental Handicap and the Human Condition.* Free Association Books, London.

Skodol, A.E., Siever, L.J. & Livesley, W.J. (2002) The borderline diagnosis II: biology, genetics, and clinical course. *Biological Psychiatry,* **51**, 951–963.

Sobsey, D. (1994) *Violence and Abuse in the Lives of People with Disabilities: The End of Silent Acceptance?* Brookes Publishing, Baltimore.

Sobsey, D. & Varnhagen, C.K. (1988) *Sexual Abuse and Exploitation of People with Disabilities.* Final Report for Child Sexual Abuse Initiative, Health and Welfare Canada.

Sobsey, D. & Varnhagen, C. (1989) Sexual abuse of people with disabilities. In: *Special Education Across Canada: Challenges for the 90s* (eds M. Csapo & L. Gougen), pp. 199–218. Centre for Human Development and Research, Vancouver.

Sobsey, D. & Varnhagen, C. (1991) Sexual abuse, assault, and exploitation of individuals with disabilities. In: *Child Sexual Abuse: Critical Perspectives on Presentation, Intervention, and Treatment* (eds C. Vagley & R.J. Thomlinson), pp. 203–216. Wall & Emerson, Toronto.

Statham, D.J., Heath, A.C., Madden, P.A., *et al.* (1998) Suicidal behaviour: an epidemiological and genetic study. *Psychological Medicine,* **28**, 839–855.

Statistics Canada (1994) *Federal-Provincial Working Group on Child and Family Services. Annual Statistical Report 1992–93 to 1994–95.* Statistics Canada, Ottawa.

Statistics Canada (2006) *Causes of Death 2003.* Statistics Canada, Ottawa.

Statistics Canada (2008) Suicides and suicide rate, by sex and by age group. Statistics Canada, Ottawa.

Sutherland, J.E., Sutherland, S.J. & Hoehns, J.D. (2003) Achieving the best outcome in treatment of depression. *Journal of Family Practice,* **53**, 118–126.

Tajfel, H. & Turner, J. (1979) An integrative theory of intergroup conflict. In: *The Social Psychology of Intergroup Relations* (eds W.G. Austin & S. Worschel), pp. 33–47. Brooks/Cole, Monterey.

Terry, D.J., Hogg, M.A. & McKimmie, B.M. (2000) Group salience, norm congruency, and mode of behavioral decision-making: the effect of group norms on attitude–behavior relations. *British Journal of Social Psychology,* **39**, 337–361.

The Peoples Law School. (2004) *Abuse of People with Disabilities: Fact Sheet.* The Peoples Law School, Vancouver. Available at http://www.publiclegaled.bc.ca/snapfiles/Abuse_Disabil._Fact_sheet.pdf (accessed 8 May 2008).

Tondo, L. (2000) *Prima del tempo. Capire e Prevenire il suicidio.* Carocci, Rome.

Tondo, L. & Baldessarini, R.J. (2001) *Suicide: Historical, Descriptive, and Epidemiological Considerations.* Available at http://www.medscape.com/viewprogram/352_pnt (accessed 2 August 2005).

United States Department of Health and Human Services (2001) *National Strategy for Suicide Prevention: Goals and Objectives for Action*. United States Department of Health and Human Services, Public Health Service, Rockville, Maryland.

Wagner, B.M. (1997) Family risk factors for child and adolescent suicide attempts. *Psychological Bulletin*, **121**, 246–298.

Wagner, B.M. & Cohen, P. (1994) Adolescent sibling differences in suicidal symptoms: the role of parent–child relationships. *Journal of Abnormal Child Psychology*, **22**, 321–337.

Westcott, H. & Jones, D. (1999) Annotation: the abuse of disabled children. *Child Psychology and Psychiatry*, **40**, 497–506.

World Health Organization (2002) *Self-Directed Violence*. Available at http://www.who.int/violence_injury_prevention/violence/world_report/factsheets/en/selfdirectedviolfacts.pdf (accessed 10 August 2005).

World Health Organization (2004) *Suicide Rates in the United States of America*. Available at http://www.who.int/mental_health/media/unitstates.pdf (accessed 16 March 2008).

Zahl, D.L. & Hawton, K. (2004) Repetition of deliberate self-harm and subsequent suicide risk: a long-term follow-up study of 11,583 patients. *British Journal of Psychiatry*, **185**, 70–75.

Zimmerman, S.L. (2002) States' spending for public welfare and their suicide rates, 1960 to 1995. What is the problem? *Journal of Nervous and Mental Disease*, **190**, 349–360.

Zung, W.W.K. (1965) A self-rating depression scale. *Archives of General Psychiatry*, **12**, 63–70.

Chapter 7

Risk of Substance Misuse

Lois Dugmore

Introduction

Substance misuse is an emotive subject, which invariably everyone has an opinion on. It is also an unspoken topic to a certain extent. When broached the majority of individuals will know someone who uses drugs or openly talks about their own drug use. Within the healthcare field it is still a subject that professionals find difficult to address. Dual diagnosis is a complex condition for which many are judgemental. It is essential in today's healthcare system to be able to clearly engage clients regarding substance misuse and be able to help them deal with the issues. In recent years the plight of pop stars and celebrities has raised the issue of substance abuse, but have drugs become more acceptable to use or does this situation act as a warning? As the availability of drugs becomes easier and street prices continue to fall (Bennetto 2006) the impact on mental health is becoming clearer (Department of Health 2002a).

In spite of the high rates of dual diagnosis, substance misuse still goes undetected within acute mental health and forensic settings. This is partly owing to the lack of training healthcare professionals receive to identify the issues and also to the lack of detection during assessment. Additionally it is because of staff concerns about how to deal with it if it is identified as an issue (Department of Health 2002b). Moreover, healthcare professionals often find it difficult to ask clients for consent for screening, as part of assessment. However, in some settings, such as forensic, screening can be part of the treatment order and therefore easier to carry out. Although screening is not the only answer it does provide a useful indicator for healthcare professionals about the individuals' substance use patterns.

When identifying the risk of substance abuse there are two elements to risk assessment:

- the actual risk of drug abuse *to* the user;
- the concerns the general public have about risk *from* substance users (Wright *et al.* 2006).

It is also important from the outset to understand that a number of individuals use substances as self-medication to cope with varying aspects of mental health, and a small percentage will actually feel mentally well by self-medicating, but for a larger percentage illicit drug use will have a negative and detrimental effect on their mental health, especially in respect of schizophrenia (Department of Health 2002b, p.8).

Within dual diagnosis there are a number of factors associated with presentation, and these include level of violence within this client group and lifestyle, which is regarded as a major contributing factor alongside drug use (Johns 1997). Another contributing factor is that a large number of drug users will use more than one drug and this multidrug use will often coexist with alcohol use, which can complicate the individuals' presentation to mental health services. To put this into context it is essential to identify those individuals receiving treatment from drug agencies, as the issues are not isolated within mental health.

The National Treatment Agency for Substance Misuse (2007a) reports that 195,464 people were in contact with specialist drug treatment in England during 2006/2007, an increase of 10% from the previous year. Among the severely mentally ill population this equates to common use of cannabis and alcohol within 33% of the population, although this is thought to be an underestimation (Department of Health 2002b).

One of the biggest conundrums facing healthcare professionals is the debate on the chicken and egg scenario – which comes first: substance misuse or mental health? Dual diagnosis guidelines (Department of Health 2002b) recognise that it does not matter which comes first, it is essential to treat the symptoms and then identify the components to meet the client's needs. The rule of thumb should be that whichever service feels it can meet the needs of the client should lead care through the co-ordination role and that both drug and mental health teams will be involved. Currently 60% of the prison population in England and Wales will have been through detoxification programmes and 70% of prisoners will present with mental health and substance use problems (Office of National Statistics 1997). To put the scale of the problem in context, figures from the National Treatment Agency for Substance Misuse (2007b) give expenditure on substance misuse at £373.3 million for 2006/2007, with an increase of 3.7% on the previous year's spend. To put the issues into perspective, legal prescribing for benzodiazepines was 20 million prescriptions in 2004/2005 (Ashton 2006).

Within forensic services individuals are more likely to have complex needs, including untreated psychoses and substance misuse issues, be from a deprived socio-economic background and have been in some form of institutional care (Prins 2005). It is essential that forensic staff are skilled in a range of therapeutic modalities for this client group. Hughes (2006) sets out in the capability framework for dual diagnosis core skills and values to address complex needs. This framework includes essential issues such as training, assessments in the workplace, service planning and needs assessment. Furthermore, the in-patient guidelines for dual diagnosis (Department of Health 2006) set down the criteria for service planning, clinical management, training of staff and management of services.

This chapter aims to outline through the exploration of policy why risk and substance misuse is an issue for all healthcare professionals. It will incorporate mental health and forensic service need for substance users with mental health issues. In the description of services, a number of the issues will have common characteristics and for specific services the provision for service will differ depending on the level of security. To fully understand the needs of the client group we need to look at the clinical components, which include dependence, substances and their management.

Dependence

According to Gelder *et al.* (2001, p.538), dependence is defined as physiological and psychological phenomena created by the continuous taking of a substance. This includes:

- a strong need to take the substance;
- development of tolerance to the substance;
- a physical withdrawal state;
- lack of ability to find alternative activity;
- being unable to concentrate on anything except the substance.

Dependence on drugs or alcohol can affect individuals' ability to perform their duties, impair or affect their attendance at work and may lead to them endangering the safety of others. Dependence on drugs or alcohol can lead to individuals using alcohol or drugs at the work place and during work hours which may affect their performance and affect others (National Treatment Agency for Substance Misuse 2004).

Most commonly used illegal or non-prescribed drugs

This section discusses the commonly used illegal or non-prescribed drugs that mental health nurses may find their clients are abusing. Drugs are classed into three categories and each carry different responses by the criminal justice services. This should be viewed as a reference section for information related to each drug. These drugs can be normally classified as follows:

Class A drugs
- Illegal to have, supply, give away or sell.
- Up to 7 years in jail.
- For supplying someone else with a class A drug you can receive life imprisonment and an unlimited fine.
- Passing drugs to friends is classed as supplying.

Class B drugs
- Illegal to possess, give away or sell.
- Up to 5 years in jail for possession.
- Up to 14 years for supplying and an unlimited fine.

Class C drugs
- Maximum penalty is 2 years in prison.
- Less serious cases will receive a warning.
- Can be arrested for carrying a small amount.
- Illegal to smoke in public.
- Illegal to drive whilst under the influence.

The information on all these drugs is taken from http://www.talktofrank. com which is a government website to support drug users, families and carers and provide information to healthcare professionals. It includes where to get help and to be able to ask questions on drugs and substance misuse.

Cannabis

Cannabis is a class C drug (see the drug classification) that can be smoked in a cigarette (spliff) with tobacco or in a pipe. It can also be injected or added to food, such as brownies, or drunk in tea. Cannabis is also known as weed, grass, skunk, black, blast, blow, Ganja, resin, hashish, herb, marijuana, sensi, hemp, backy or zero. There are two types of cannabis:

1. Hash – which is a black/brown lump made from the resin of the plant and the grass is the dried leaves from the plant;
2. Sinsemillia – which is less common and is a bud grown in the absence of male plants and has no seeds.

The current cost of cannabis is estimated at £30–80 per ounce. Table 7.1 summarises the effects and risk factors of cannabis.

Heroin

Heroin is a class A drug that is an opiate. It is a white powder but when cut with other substances can be brownish, white or brown. Heroin can be smoked, snorted, or injected when dissolved in water. Heroin is also known

Table 7.1   The effects and risk factors of cannabis.

Effects	Risk factors
• Gives a sedative effect • People feel calm • Can cause nausea • Causes the giggles • Gives a feeling of hunger (known as the 'munchies') • Affects co-ordination • Causes anxiety, paranoia, suspicion and panic	• Can be problematic for asthma suffers • Increases blood pressure • Suggested link with cannabis and mental health issues. • Will increase paranoia for those with existing mental health issues • Possible dependency • Reduces male sperm count and suppresses ovulation in women • Results in difficulty motivating oneself • Makes user feel tired and have difficulty concentrating

Table 7.2   The effects and risk factors of heroin.

Effects	Risk factors
• Slows down body function and stops pain • Gives a rush after a few minutes of taking it • Smaller doses give a feeling of well being • Larger doses make the individual feel tired and sleepy • Takes a longer period of time to become addicted • Strong psychological and physical dependence after a period of time	• Deaths from overdose • Can cause respiratory failure or coma with large doses • Overdose more likely when used with alcohol or benzodiazepines • Vein damage when injected (can lead to gangrene on rare occasions) • Risk of blood-borne infections, e.g. hepatitis B and C, HIV/AIDS from sharing equipment

as brown, skag, H gear, smack or horse. The current cost is estimated at £30–100 per gram. Table 7.2 summarises the effects and risk factors of heroin.

Stimulant drugs including cocaine, crack cocaine, amphetamines, MDMA and LSD

Cocaine
Cocaine is a class A drug which is also known as coke, Charlie, C, white lines and base. It is a white powder that is usually divided in lines. The

Table 7.3   The effects and risk factors of cocaine.

Effects	Risk factors
• Cocaine is very addictive • Cocaine is a stimulant so makes people feel confident • Effect is immediate and lasts between 20 and 30 minutes • Makes a person feel alive, excited, wide-awake • Reduces appetite • Leads to rapid tolerance • Person feels restless, irritable and anxious • Reduces tiredness • Gives ability to dance, and feel able to carry on for a longer period of time • Results in hallucinations, paranoia and mood swings • Leads to aggression and violence • Causes nausea and vomiting • Results in tiredness and depression • Regular users look excited but nervous • Heavy users find it difficult to sleep	• When using very high does there have been deaths associated with heart failure or respiratory arrest, although this is rare. • Regular use of cocaine may lead to physical and psychological dependence within a relatively short period of use • Overdose associated when mixed with other drugs such as heroin, barbiturates or alcohol • In existing high blood pressure and heart conditions, cocaine can increase blood pressure and exacerbate symptoms • High dosage can lead to seizure or fits • Damages septum in nose through snorting cocaine • Can cause breathing difficulties • Can cause panic attacks • High cost of the drug because after a short period of time more of the drug is required to maintain the high • Leads to debt problems • Strong link to crime due to stealing or other criminal behaviour to fund the habit • Reduces libido • Crack cocaine (see below) can increase mental health symptoms • Crack cocaine (see below) is associated with premature labour in pregnant users, miscarriage, smaller babies and low birth weight, and may cause birth abnormalities. Babies show withdrawal symptoms on birth • Exacerbates existing mental health issues • Easier to overdose when injecting

method of use is normally through snorting up the nose, but it can be smoked or made into a solution and injected. The current estimated cost per gram is £35–65. Table 7.3 summarises the effects and risk factors of cocaine.

Crack cocaine

'Crack' is a class A drug which is a derivative of cocaine mixed with baking soda and water, and is sold in small 'rocks' about the size of a small pea. It is also known as rocks, stones, pebbles, wash, freebase, crack or base. Crack is usually smoked using a crack pipe, glass tube or plastic bottle, in foil or tin can, but can also be injected. The current cost is estimated at £10–25 per rock. Table 7.4 summarises the effects and risk factors of crack cocaine.

Amphetamine (MDA, methylenedioxy-amphetamine/MDEA, methyl diethanol amine)

Amphetamine is a class B drug, unless it is prepared for injection when it becomes a class A drug. It is also known as phet, sulphate, billy, whiz, sulph, paste dexamphetamine, dexies or base. The current cost is estimated at £8–12 a wrap. Amphetamine is an off-white or pinkish powder, sometimes made into tablets. It is swallowed, snorted, injected or smoked. Table 7.5 summarises the effects and risk factors of amphetamine.

Ecstasy (MDMA, methylenedioxymethamphetamine)

Ecstasy is a class A drug which is sold in tablet form and comes in many colours and some have pictures imprinted on them. It is also known as E, pills, brownies, burgers, disco biscuits, rolex's, dolphins or XTC. The current cost is estimated at £2–8 per pill. Table 7.6 summarises the effects and risk factors of ecstasy.

LSD

LSD is a class A drug that is sold as small squares of paper, sometimes with pictures on them. They are taken orally. It is also known as acid, cheer, dots, drop, flash, hawk, L, liquid acid, lucy, micro dot, paper mushrooms, stars, tab, trips or tripper. The current cost is estimated at £1–5 a tablet. Table 7.7 summarises the effects and risk factors of LSD.

Steroids

Steroids are a class C drug that is also known as roids. However, this name can vary around the country. Steroids are purchased as tablets or liquid for injecting. They are used to improve body image or for sports people to improve performance. The current estimated cost is around £3 a score. Table 7.8 summarises the effects and risk factors of steroids.

Table 7.4   The effects and risk factors of crack cocaine.

Effects	Risk factors
• Same short-acting effects as cocaine but much more addictive • Effect is immediate and lasts between 2 and 10 minutes • Makes a person feel alive, excited, confident, lively, wide-awake • Reduces appetite • Leads to rapid tolerance • Person feels restless, irritable and anxious. • Leads to increased sensitivity to anaesthetic • Reduces tiredness • After 20 minutes, cravings for more start • Results in hallucinations, paranoia and mood swings • Leads to aggression and violence • Causes nausea and vomiting • Causes tiredness and depression • Regular users look excited but nervous • Heavy users find it difficult to sleep • Leads to severe depression in withdrawal • Has associated stress, anxiety and effect on mental health • Agitates delirium and paranoid psychoses	• Although rare there have been deaths from overdose • High doses can increase temperature, convulsions and respiratory arrest • Combining alcohol with cocaine can cause a chemical reaction producing coca-ethylene which increases cocaine's euphoric effects, while potentially increasing the risk of sudden death • Regular use of crack may lead to physical and psychological dependence within a relatively short period of use • Existing high blood pressure and heart conditions can be exacerbated • High dosage can lead to seizure or fits • Can cause breathing difficulties • Can cause panic attacks • High cost of drug because after a short period of time more of the drug is required to maintain the high • Leads to debt problems • Strong link to crime due to funding the habit • Reduces libido • Crack can increase mental health symptoms • Crack is associated with premature labour in pregnant users, miscarriage, smaller babies and low birth weight, and may cause birth abnormalities. Babies show withdrawal symptoms on birth • Stimulants can prolong the duration of psychotic illness

Table 7.5 The effects and risk factors of amphetamine.

Effects	Risk factors
• Effects start about 30 minutes after ingestion but can last for 6 hours • Makes the individual feel wide awake, excited and talkative • Supplies energy to dance for hours • Person cannot keep still or sleep • Results in irritability and depression that can last for days on coming down from the high • Person sniffs a lot • Results in hallucinations and panic	• There have been deaths associated with amphetamine use • Known to affect the heart and not suggested for individuals with high blood pressure • Deaths have been associated with mixed amphetamines with alcohol or antidepressants • Affects the immune system • Damages veins of injecting users • Easy to overdose if injecting

Table 7.6 The effects and risk factors of ecstasy.

Effects	Risk factors
• Takes 30 minutes to work and lasts 3–6 hours • Gives a buzz that makes the person feel very awake • Person can dance for hours without feeling tired • Brings out intensity in sounds and colours • Makes emotions more intense • Makes people more sociable and talk a lot • Dilates pupils and tightens jaw muscles	• Short-term anxiety • Panic attack, confusion • First time epileptic fits and paranoia • Depression, personality change and memory loss with long-term use • 200 deaths since 1996 due to loss of body temperature control or heart failure • Linked to kidney liver and heart problems • Paranoia and depression • Dehydration • Drinking too much water • More likely to get colds, flu and sore throats • Problematic for anyone with asthma, high blood pressure or a heart condition

Table 7.7   The effects and risk factors of LSD.

Effects	Risk factors
• Takes up to 2 hours to work • Can last up to 12 hours • Trips can be fun or build on fears and paranoia • Accentuates colour senses • Speeds up movement and time • Can slow down movement and time • Sound, colour and objects can be distorted • Results in panic and confusion • No addictive properties	• Interaction with existing mental health issues • Bad trips can be frightening • Flashbacks can occur weeks/months after the last time LSD was used • Accidents can occur when using acid (e.g. running away from visions into traffic)

Table 7.8   The effects and risk factors of steroids.

Effects	Risk factors
• May cause aggression • Enables sports enthusiasts to train for longer • Builds body mass • Person recovers quickly from excessive exercise routines	• Not physically addictive but can be psychologically dependent • Withdrawal can cause lethargy and depression • Can cause aggression • For younger users can affect growth • With injecting can cause vein damage and risk of hepatitis/HIV when sharing equipment • Male erection problems and growth of breasts • Can develop acne • Females may develop facial hair, experience voice changes, menstrual problems • Can cause depression • Can cause paranoia • Risk of high blood pressure, liver failure, stroke or heart failure

Alcohol

Alcohol is a socially acceptable substance and is frequently used for social-isation and entertainment. Alcohol use is not limited to any psychiatric dis-order, but is frequently found as a presenting factor in suicide, self-harm and acute confusion presentations at accident and emergency departments (Department of Health 2002a). Psychiatric disorders fall into four categories:

- intoxication phenomena;
- withdrawal phenomena;
- toxic or nutritional disorders;
- associated psychiatric disorders

(Gelder *at al.* 2001).

Alcohol is also used alongside other drugs, both illegal and prescribed. Alcohol dependence will build up over a period of time. In terms of safe drinking levels the government recommends specific units per week: 21 for men and 14 for women. However, there has been confusion as to what a unit means and there are other mitigating factors such as drug use.

Ketamine

Ketamine is a class C drug that is also known as green, K, special K or vitamin K. It can be bought in tablet, powder or liquid form. Ketamine can be snorted, swallowed or injected. Table 7.9 summarises the effects and risk factors of ketamine.

Table 7.9 The effects and risk factors of ketamine.

Effects	Risk factors
<ul><li>Causes perceptual changes</li><li>Trip can last for a few hours</li><li>Out of body experience</li><li>Physically unable to move whilst under the influence</li></ul>	<ul><li>Likely to incur injury because unable to feel pain</li><li>Psychological dependence but not physical</li><li>Interacts with depressant drugs and alcohol</li><li>Leads to panic attacks</li><li>Causes depression</li><li>Exacerbates mental health systems</li><li>Death can result from inhaling vomit</li></ul>

Table 7.10   The effects and risk factors of khat.

Effects	Risk factors
<ul><li>Is a stimulant</li><li>Person feels more alert and talkative</li><li>Reduces appetite</li><li>Induces a feeling of calm</li></ul>	<ul><li>Leads to insomnia</li><li>Impotence</li><li>Heart problems</li><li>Anxiety and aggression</li><li>Irritability</li><li>Can make existing mental health problems worse</li></ul>

Khat

Khat is not an illegal drug in the UK. It is also known as quat, qat, qaadka or chat. A leaf is chewed over a period of time. It is known to be used within the Somali population in the UK. A small bunch of leaves costs around £4. Table 7.10 summarises the effects and risk factors of khat.

Benzodiazepines

Benzodiazepines are a class C drug if not prescribed by a general practitioner and are available as tablets, capsules, injectables or suppositories. They are also known as jellies, benxos, eggs, norries, rugby balls, vallies, moggles, mazzies, roofies or downers. The estimated cost is £1 per capsule. Table 7.11 summarises the effects and risk factors of benzodiazepines.

Table 7.11   The effects and risk factors of benzodiazepines.

Effects	Risk factors
<ul><li>Have sedative effects</li><li>Relieve tension and anxiety</li><li>Can cause short-term forgetfulness</li></ul>	<ul><li>Can cause both physical and psychological dependence</li><li>Increased doses needed due to tolerance</li><li>Depressant can lead to overdose if mixed with alcohol</li><li>Crushing tablets to inject causes vein problems</li><li>Withdrawal causes headache, nausea, anxiety and confusion</li><li>Causes panic attacks on withdrawal</li><li>Rohypnol linked to sex crimes. Causes paralysis of victim and victim being both unaware and unable to stop assault or rape</li></ul>

Table 7.12 The effects and risk factors of crystal meth.

Effects	Risk factors
• Causes exhilaration and increased arousal • Results in higher energy levels • Reduced tiredness • Reduced appetite • Intense rush that lasts for 4–12 hours	• Leads to agitation • Paranoia • Confusion and violence • Known to be very addictive – both psychological and physical dependence • Widely reported from America is crystal meth-induced psychosis • Death can occur related to overdose, stroke, gastrointestinal disorders • Risks associated with injecting • Can result in increased libido and risky sexual behaviour

Crystal meth

Crystal meth is a class B drug that is also known as ice, glass, Christine, yaba, crazy medicine or methamphetamine. It can be found in tablet, powder or crystalline form and can be snorted, taken orally, smoked or injected. The estimated cost is not clear as its use in the UK is rare, but it is at epidemic proportions in many states in the USA. Table 7.12 summarises the effects and risk factors of crystal meth.

Mixing drugs

Mixing drugs is common practice among abusers. Alcohol and drugs of any kind are frequently used together. Alcohol will cause a depressive effect on the drug use. A further common mixing of drugs is by injecting heroin and cocaine together, which is called 'speed balling' or 'curry and chips'. Drug services have seen an increasing number of service users and there have been a number of deaths associated with this practice. Users describe the effects of a combined stimulant and sedative as feeling the rush of crack while the heroin takes the edge off coming down from the drug. The average cost of a speed ball is £20. Bennetto (2006) considers that people who 'speed ball' are three times more likely to have a conviction as they can spend up to £500 a week in acquiring the drugs.

Policy

Traditionally services have been developed based on individual need and have not combined shared care. The *Dual Diagnosis Good Practice Guide* (Department of Health 2002b) recommends that services provide integrated care for individuals who have both mental health problems and substance misuse. It places the emphasis on mental health services to ensure that clients can access substance misuse services. Substance misuse includes all drugs – both licit and illicit. It also includes alcohol use. It is also worth considering the use of tobacco and caffeine when considering drug use, as a number of clients will also be dependent on these substances and may be involved with their substance use. The term dual diagnosis as described by the Department of Health (2002b) covers a wide range of mental health and substance misuse issues, which broadly include:

- a primary psychiatric illness precipitating or leading to substance misuse;
- substance misuse worsening or altering the course of psychiatric illness;
- intoxication and/or substance dependence leading to psychological symptoms;
- substance misuse and/or withdrawal leading to psychiatric symptoms or illnesses.

Dual diagnosis for many has been a contentious issue, and the issues of service provision have been much debated. It is agreed through the *Dual Diagnosis Good Practice Guide* (Department of Health 2002b) for England that care should remain within mainstream mental health services. It recommends:

'. . . a framework within which staff can strengthen services so that they have the skills and organisation to tackle this demanding area of work' (p.3).

It has one key message:

'. . . that substance misuse is already part of mainstream mental health services and this is the right place for skills and services to be' (p.3).

The focus of attention should, therefore, be on training healthcare professionals to work with clients presenting with both mental health and substance misuse issues. One of the main concerns has been around the development of skills for healthcare professionals, and how to train them to work with clients who are using illicit substances or alcohol. Integrated treatment in the UK can be delivered by existing mental health services following training and with close liaison and joint working will substance misuse services. Training and education regarding dual diagnosis and substance misuse has played a small role in education programmes for mental health staff and this needs to be addressed through nurse training.

Within the *Dual Diagnosis Good Practice Guide* (Department of Health 2002b) the focus is on mental health and substance misuse, and it reiterates the policy context set by the *Mental Health National Service Framework* (Department of Health 1999) and *Tackling Drugs Together to Build a Better Britain* (Department of Health 1998), which demonstrate the need to work jointly to manage the issues. The *Dual Diagnosis Good Practice Guide* places responsibility for implementation of service improvement jointly with National Service Framework Implementation Teams and acute mental health services. There is also a role for Drug Action Teams via the National Treatment Agency for Substance Misuse (2002) *Models of Care* document, which sets out a national framework for the commissioning of treatment for adult drug misusers in England, although similar models apply to other parts of the United Kingdom and the world based on joint working, to ensure drug users have access to drug services, and attention should be given to those with co-occurring disorders. It is the Drug Action Teams' role to develop strategies based on local need and also to implement the model of care to meet the needs of drug users. The framework model is based on a four-tier model to access services.

The *Dual Diagnosis Good Practice Guide* (Department of Health 2002b) highlights the importance of related guidelines on drug misuse and dependence and those on models of care for substance misuse services. It considers the evidence base in assessment and treatment, illustrating this with examples of good practice.

Building Bridges: A Guide to Arrangements for Inter-Agency Working for the Care and Protection of Severely Mentally Ill People (Department of Health 1996) 10 years ago prioritised the need to ensure close working links between community mental health teams and community drug teams to ensure collaborative working practices. The aim was to ensure that the care programme process (Department of Health 1990) was implemented using a collaborative approach, and when used in conjunction with the *Dual Diagnosis Good Practice Guide* (Department of Health 2002b) it can provide a framework within which staff can strengthen services.

The 10-year strategy for substance misuse (Department of Health 1998) identifies significant risks for young people using substances being related to psychological problems. *Safer Services: Report of the National Confidential Inquiry into Suicide and Homicide by People with Mental Illness* (Appleby *et al.* 1999) identifies the need to make provision for dual diagnosis clients within mainstream services. The literature clearly recognises the links between dual diagnosis and the criminal justice system (Phillips 2000) and the need for focused services. National policy also supports the use of assertive outreach models and teams (Department of Health 1999).

Publications and policies incorporated within a local strategy should include:

- the Misuse of Drugs Act (1971);
- the *Mental Health National Service Framework* (Department of Health 1999);
- *The NHS Plan* (Department of Health 2000);
- *The Essence of Care: Patient-Focused Benchmarking for Health Care Practitioners* (Department of Health 2001a);
- National Institute for Health and Clinical Excellence (NICE) guidelines;
- clinical governance and performance frameworks;
- Commission for Health Improvements (CHI) reports, Audit reports and Social Services Inspectorate reports;
- patient surveys;
- National Institute for Mental Health in England (NIMHE) guidelines;
- national inquiries;
- *Dual Diagnosis Good Practice Guide* (Department of Health 2002b);
- *The National Service Framework for Mental Health – Five Years On* (Department of Health 2004).

Local primary care, mental health, criminal justice and substance misuse services in the statutory, voluntary and independent sectors need to work together with service users/carers to explore both mental health and substance misuse services to meet individual needs. Between 33 and 50% of individuals accessing mental health services will have a co-occurring substance misuse problem (Department of Health 2002a). Phillips (2000) recognises the need for an effective psychiatric nursing response to assessment and joint clinical management. He also brings attention to the increased rates of violence in dual diagnosis. *The National Confidential Inquiry into Suicide and Homicide* (Department of Health 2001b) showed that at least half of all suicides were associated with dual diagnosis.

Issues associated with substance misuse and mental health

Profile of service user group

People with a dual diagnosis aged between 18 and 65 years are more vulnerable than those presenting with a single diagnosis. Their prognosis is considered more unpredictable, with high levels of service use and disengagement. They are a high user of in-patient beds and community facilities. According to the Department of Health (2002a) they are also more likely to:

- have a history of childhood abuse (sexual/physical);
- have increased suicide risk or self-harm risk;
- have severe mental health problems;
- be homeless or in unsuitable housing;
- be victims of crime;
- be in contact with the criminal justice system;
- have a history of family problems;
- disengage with services and be non-compliant with treatment;
- abscond from in-patient facilities;
- experience higher levels of violence;
- have physical health problems related to neglect and drug/alcohol use;
- not always receive appropriate care;
- experience post traumatic stress/trauma;
- have longer and more frequent hospital admissions;
- experience intense delusional ideation;
- find prescribed drugs less effective;
- be non compliant with treatment and medication;
- be difficult to diagnose;
- experience frequent crisis presentations.

On top of this they will probably be known to a range of services including:

- Accident and Emergency;
- primary care;
- the homeless service;
- the drug/alcohol team;
- prisons;
- hostels;
- social services;
- GPs;
- child protection;
- carer support services;
- voluntary sector services;
- mental health services.

Alexander and Haugland (2000) published a major report examining mental health and substance misuse strategies. The report considered research evidence and clinical studies from the USA. The authors of this report view the terms dual diagnosis and co-morbidity as a reflection of the

continuing lack of understanding and ambiguity of these complex presentations. It is clear that to meet the needs of this client group it is essential to
complete a comprehensive assessment that incorporates substance use, risk
and mental health. Alexander and Haugland identified services such as
assertive community treatment as providing effective care for those with a
co-occurring disorder. They also recognised that within forensic services
clients do well until the point of release, when problems occur with follow-
up. Case study 1 in Box 7.1 demonstrates the need for collaborative working with other services with a shared care plan.

Box 7.1   Case study 1: Sue

Sue is a 35-year-old white British female. She has used cannabis (skunk
and resin), heroin, amphetamines, cocaine, crack cocaine, alcohol, tobacco and
caffeine. Sue has overcome all drugs except alcohol and occasional cannabis
use, but in the past has used various methods including injecting, ingestion,
smoking, snorting and chasing.

She has a diagnosis of personality disorder with psychotic features and was
previously diagnosed with paranoid schizophrenia. She has a history of self-harm
including overdose, cutting and using substances and alcohol in particular to
cope. She has a long history of childhood sexual abuse and has been abused
and raped as an adult. Sue has issues with sexuality and has been helped by
housing support workers through two court cases related to the rape charges.
Sue has been involved with mental health services since the age of 15 and in
touch with drug services from the age of 18.

Sue has a history of violence and responds in a violent manner when feeling
vulnerable. She has been a victim of assault. Sue develops relationships with
individuals with violent histories and has been a victim of assault by partners and
raped within these relationships. There is a past history of violence to figures
of authority and care workers. Sue has been made homeless on a number of
occasions. When experiencing elements of paranoia Sue will become isolated
and feels unable to seek help. Sue has a history of abusing alcohol and substance
misuse at times of stress. She also has epilepsy and experiences fits when not
taking medication. Sue is frequently non-compliant with medication. She has no
forensic history.

Sue is currently receiving care via the following services:

- housing association with housing worker to help with everyday tasks;
- dual diagnosis nurse to talk about harm minimisation and work on relapse
  prevention;
- rape crisis councillor to deal with issues related to previous assaults;
- community mental health nurse for her depot;
- outpatient services for epilepsy;
- day services for anger management.

The following risk factors can be identified:

- risk of violence from partners;
- risk of violence to workers;
- risk of self-harm – overdose and cutting;
- risk from drug and alcohol relapse;
- physical risk when epilepsy not controlled;
- non-compliance with medication;
- has previous history of being homeless;
- family contact due to abuse issues within the family;
- has in the past been banned from mental health units because of levels of aggression.

Although Sue receives a comprehensive package of care, she feels at times overwhelmed by the number of individuals seeing her and would prefer to have one worker to discuss everything. The team meet every month to discuss current issues; these meetings include Sue and anyone she feels she would like to be there. A care plan is agreed and a copy given to all those involved including Sue. Within this system Sue has access to telephone support 24 hours a day regarding her drug/alcohol use. Her CPN monitors her medication and mental health and assists her with visits to the outpatient consultant clinic. Sue accesses the voluntary sector for anger management and finds this very helpful. The dual diagnosis nurse monitors drug/alcohol issues and works with relapse prevention and cravings.

Assessment

A comprehensive mental health and substance misuse assessment is fundamental to fully understand and treat a client who both uses substances and experiences mental health difficulties. This assessment may take a considerable period of time to ensure it is comprehensive.

There are a number of recognised drug and alcohol assessment tools available including:

- Cage Alcohol Screening Tool (CAGE) (Ewing 1984);
- Michigan Alcohol Screening Tool (MAST) (Selzer 1971);
- Drug Abuse Screening Tool (DAST) (Gavin *et al.* 1989);
- Clinical Drug Use Scale (CDUS) (Drake *et al.* 1989);
- Substance Abuse Treatment Scale (SATS) (McHugo *et al.* 1995);
- Leeds Dependence Questionnaire (LDQ) (Raistrick *et al.* 1994);
- Stages of change – readiness to change ruler (Miller and Rollnick 1998).

The assessment should consider:

- full drug/alcohol history;
- age at first use;
- methods of use;
- drugs tried;
- persons used with (friends/family/alone);
- current financial situation (debts/loans/how they finance drugs);
- full mental health history;
- forensic history (cautions/convictions/outstanding court cases);
- previous treatment (counselling/detoxification);
- urine screening/saliva screening.

When working with clients, to enable staff to work with their client on his or her drug/alcohol use and to monitor the effects of the drug/alcohol on the client's mental health, it is essential to use recognised models to monitor change and improvement. Within the cycle of change there are five stages an individual will go through when thinking about stopping substance use (Prochaska and DiClemente 1983):

1. Pre-contemplation – where the person does not believe he/she has a problem.
2. Contemplation – where the person has begun to think it may be an issue and wants to change.
3. Preparation – where the person plans how he or she will make the changes and set goals.
4. Action – where the individual makes the changes and works towards goals.
5. Maintenance – where the person keeps up the changes he/she has made.

It will also allow clients to access drug/alcohol treatment by accepting they have a problem. This will be different in forensic settings where it is standard practice to screen as part of care.

Urine or saliva screening is a very contentious issue within both mental health and forensic settings. When requesting that a client be screened, the approach taken by the staff member is crucial; it should always be seen as a positive experience. It should be used as a means to allow staff to help the client and be clear what the client has been taking. Clients at times do not know what they have been taking because of what they have taken or because they have purchased something that is not what they requested. Screening should be used to enable staff to monitor and ensure the client receives the right type of medication. It will enable staff to work with their clients on their drug/alcohol use and to monitor the effects of the drug/alcohol on clients' mental health. Within mental health settings consent needs to be sought from the client for screening. It is also worth considering the method of screening, as urine screening needs to be supervised and this can be seen as degrading. There is also the option of saliva screening which is less invasive and can be carried out as part of an assessment. Hair and blood samples can also be used, but although very effective they are not cost efficient.

Following assessment the plan should include such issues as:

- problems of substance misuse;
- methods of use;
- specific complex issues;
- increased risk of risky behaviours;
- assessment;
- detox;
- treatment;
- risk;
- interventions;
- management;
- the nurse–patient relationship;
- gender;
- culture;
- planning for relapse prevention/relapse.

Care pathways

Integrated care pathways are based on the current best evidence gained from systematic reviews (Health Services and Utilization and Research Council 2001) as well as information from clinical teams and clients. The advantages are that they bring about quality improvement and are able to track key indicators and processes that look at how the client's care can be improved. To achieve a coordinated approach to care pathways there needs to be an agreed definition and all relevant agencies need to be signed up to the process and involved in clinical governance forums. This will ensure that care is delivered directly and efficiently to the client, and provides an evaluation process and a team approach. An integrated care pathway will draw together a team of professionals who will sign up to a specific care pathway that meets the needs of the individual client group in a systematic way. The integrated care pathway should:

- result in opportunities for improving care delivery;
- enhance multidisciplinary planning and problem solving;

- allow clients and carers to be part of the process;
- provide consistent care;
- ensure interventions are appropriate;
- standardise practice;
- improve outcomes;
- ensure continuity and discharge planning;
- promote good communication;
- be linked to clinical governance;
- be agreed by stakeholder group.

A care pathway for local services across the health and social care community needs to be owned by those implementing it. Care pathways need to be underpinned by shared care protocols and treatment protocols that promote appropriate transfer between services, safe discharge and mechanisms for re-referral. In line with joint working, confidentiality protocols and information-sharing protocols need to be agreed between all agencies because of the complexity of organisations and the client group. The needs of people with a dual diagnosis should be addressed holistically – with a designated care co-ordinator in the relevant team and by better integration of existing services and providing joint care services where both mental health and drug/alcohol services co-work with a client (see Figure 7.1 for an example of a care pathway).

Within the care pathways there should be development of core assessment and care protocols – for substance misuse, mental health and learning disability, including greater consistency in retaining case responsibility and where necessary transferring people's care between teams. There should be a review of the guidelines and policies for drug dealing/drug misuse in residential, forensic and ward settings and in relation to dealing with challenging behaviours that can be associated with substance misuse, the latter to include maximising assistance to staff from other team colleagues. It is essential to have a consistent approach to enable clients to be able to ask for and to accept help with drug/alcohol use.

Policies need to incorporate legal issues related to drug use and to ensure that other clients within treatment areas are protected. There need to be improvements made in relation to links/liaison between secondary care teams – each current team in ward, community and forensic (mental health, learning disability, substance misuse, etc.) settings should be integrated with accident and emergency services, prison services and primary care to ensure a consistent approach to care. There should be improved therapeutic follow-up following discharge from the forensic setting, acute in-patient mental healthcare, inpatient detoxification, streamlining of the 'community care' assessment procedure and improved support/liaison in the event of relapse. In forensic settings the follow-up needs to be clearly defined, as the

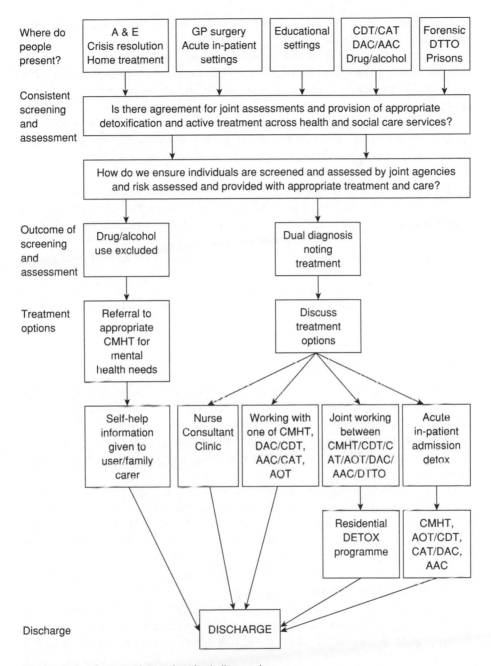

Figure 7.1 Care pathway for dual diagnosis.
Abbreviations: A & E (Accident and Emergency); GP (General Practitioner); CDT
(Community Drug Team); CAT (Community Alcohol Team); DAC (Drug Advice Centre); AAC
(Alcohol Advice Centre); DTTO (Drug Testing Treatment Order); AOT (Assertive Outreach
Team); CMHT (Community Mental Health Team); DETOX (Detoxification).

issues relating to re-offending and its relationship to drug and alcohol use need to be followed-up.

Substance misuse and mental health problems are now a current issue for mental health professionals. When working in a mental health setting staff need to be proactive and employ a variety of skills to engage the dual diagnosis population. This includes addressing social exclusion. To address social exclusion, access to services needs to be made available to marginalised groups; this can be achieved by language translations, picture adverts for those with reading issues and acceptance of differences, and also by outreach services going into communities and discussing and sharing information. Risk assessment is a major feature in the care of individuals with mental health issues. Mental health professionals are responsible for ensuring that a comprehensive risk assessment is carried out and that assessment associates all elements of risk. Risk cannot just be seen as an incident of harm to others. There are a number of risks associated with an individual that require thorough assessment. These include issues around drug use and safe practices in regard to injecting, quantity of substances used following a break in drug use and the risk of overdose. Care plans need to incorporate risk management to help key workers manage risk.

Drug-induced psychosis

Co-morbid conditions despite recent interest have not been fully understood. Drug-induced psychosis is not fully understood and can lead to difficulties in treatment and conflict within the mental health system because of the needs of the client group and difficulty in diagnostic distinctions. Table 7.13 shows the drugs causing psychosis which should be considered.

Drug-induced psychosis is more likely to be diagnosed in Afro-Caribbean clients (Department of Health 2005). This is often based on prejudice and cultural use of drugs. One of the biggest barriers to treatment is stereotyping, which can lead to inappropriate treatment and longer admissions. There is a higher incidence of a diagnosis of psychosis being made if a client declares that he/she is using cannabis (Department of Health 2005). Individuals presenting with mental health problems and substance misuse are often turned away and left to address their drug problem first. This can be an issue as substances can cause a psychosis lasting up to 30 days after initial drug use whether or not they have stated drug use.

Drugs or alcohol can be used as reason not to admit. It is crucial to provide general supportive measures, based on reassurance and providing an environment in which it is possible to reduce stimuli and provide an area in which the client can feel safe. One of the key features to bear

Table 7.13 Drugs causing psychosis – effects and risk factors.

Cocaine	Cannabis – paranoid psychoses
• Delusions, e.g. parasitic infestation • Paranoia • Aggression	• Linked to schizophrenia-type behaviours • 2.5 times greater risk of psychoses in cannabis users and six times greater risk in heavy users • Data suggest risk factor in the development of schizophrenia for those with predisposed features • Indolence • Apathy • Bizarre behaviour • Violence • Panic
Amphetamines	**Lysergic acid diethylamide (LSD)**

• Likened to schizophrenia-type syndrome with high doses of drug
• Repetitive behaviour, e.g. constant tidying
• Features include:
  ○ Persecutory delusions
  ○ Auditory/visual hallucinations
  ○ Hostile/dangerous behaviour
  ○ Aggression
• Effects usually subside in a week after stopping drug but can go on for up to 6 months
	• Secondary paranoia
	• Distorts time, colour, sound, movement and distance
	• Accidents
	• Homicide
	• Self-harm
	• Flashbacks
	• Visual hallucinations with great vividness
	• Unearthing of schizophrenic tendencies
	• Works on seratonin and mimics 5-hydroxytriptamine

in mind is that psychosis, however caused, is serious and disabling and for the individual to remain safe and without risk it is important to treat the psychosis. Whatever the cause, the symptoms need to be treated. Clients presenting following drug use are highly likely to have predisposing factors for psychosis. There are a substantial number of case reports of cannabis-induced psychoses. Schizophrenic patients who continue to use cannabis respond poorly to neuroleptic drugs, experience more psychotic symptoms, have higher rates of continuous hallucinations and delusions, and more hospitalisations (Drake *et al.* 1998). Drug abusers have higher prevalence of hallucinations, delusions, positive symptoms, poorer compliance and a higher relapse rate (Department of Health 2002a). However, the jury is still out in relation to:

- treat the symptoms, don't look for the cause;
- look for self-medication issues;
- family histories;
- the chicken or egg – who cares!

It is important to look at how clients present and not necessarily what they are telling us. It is important to treat a psychosis no matter how it has manifested itself because of the implications to self harm and distress related to hearing voices and seeing images.

Engagement

Engagement is the first step to encouraging a client into the treatment process. It will depend on the therapeutic relationship between the staff and client. Applying a non-judgmental approach and understanding the client's experiences will assist in the process. With this client group it is important to meet the needs that present now and accept that abstinence may be a long way down the road. For now, safer injecting is a good starting point. Helping clients to deal with their daily living, housing, clothing and food may be more effective in enabling them to change their patterns. When identifying the needs of forensic clients, consideration needs to be given to expertise in court diversion to engage clients before prison. In prisons the development of in-reach workers who can work directly with clients with a dual diagnosis is essential in engaging clients.

Treatment options

One of the key indicators of success is that clients are able to accept that they have a problem. Secondly, they will need to want to do something about it. With alcohol use, early detection has proven to be an indicator of success, and a study by Chick and Cantwell (1994) demonstrates that early intervention on a medical basis can lead to the reduction of alcohol use. Motivation to change is a key factor in successful drug cessation. Miller and Rollnick (2002) describe motivational interviewing as a key way of engaging drug and alcohol clients in working through issues by providing a model that is based on helping clients to effect change and enabling client responsibility for change.

Prescribing

For some clients the option of giving up drugs seems unattainable. In these cases, based on harm minimisation, substitute prescribing may be considered (Gelder *et al.* 2001). The clinician will prescribe a less addictive drug, e.g. methadone or buprenorphine can be prescribed as a heroin substitute. This is known as maintenance therapy, and is provided alongside counselling and help with social problems including housing. The aim is to engage clients in the process of beginning to contemplate withdrawal. The rationale is to enable the client to stop using street drugs and the lifestyle involved in maintaining illicit drug use, for example theft. Maintenance therapy is predominantly used in opioid (heroin, morphine, codeine) addiction. This is usually provided in oral form in order to withdraw from injecting, but for some clients it may be necessary to prescribe an injectable form for a short period of time. The aim is also to reduce harm to the individual by engaging him or her in services and provide education on safer injection and safe sex practices. Injectable dexamphetamine prescribing may also be considered for the same reasons for intravenous amphetamine users.

Cue exposure

Cue exposure is a treatment technique that identifies issues related to tolerance, withdrawal and cravings relating to drugs and alcohol. Cue exposure works to change the client's approach to cravings (Eliany and Rush 1992). When working with drug and alcohol users the aim is to identify and work with the cues that expose the client to using (e.g. expose a crack cocaine user to rocks or an alcohol user to a glass of wine). The aim is to reduce the desire to use. Cue exposure aims to reduce the desire to use by finding out what the cues for use are and to reduce the cues. This method provides the opportunity to practise coping responses (e.g. relaxation). In reality it can increase self-efficacy, which will increase the likelihood that the response will be utilised in future. Cue exposure is realistic in that the methodology recognises that it is impossible to avoid drug-/alcohol-related cues and it is better to prepare patients to handle these cues outside of treatment to real life, including the circumstances, paraphernalia and emotions/feelings related to their drug use. Sessions are usually for a set period of around 10–12 weeks, each lasting approximately 1 hour. To be able to identify cues, equipment for each session will be required and these may include:

- photographs;
- injecting equipment;

- meeting places, such as a public house ('pub');
- current cues;
- methods of control.

Detoxification

Detoxification can take place in a number of settings including:

- the client's home;
- in-patient stand-alone hospital units;
- private drug units;
- acute medical wards;
- psychiatric wards;
- on occasions, residential rehabilitation units.

The aim of admission for detoxification is to help clients who have either failed detoxification at home or been unable to abstain from substances. In terms of detoxification it can be completed rapidly on an in-patient basis. In-patient detoxification can provide a safety net for clients and provide time to re-evaluate life and their attitude to substances. According to Day (2005), admission should provide:

- assessment of the level of dependence;
- stabilising drug use;
- stabilising drug use leading to detoxification from opioids, barbiturates, benzodiazepines or other sedative hypnotics;
- management of both drug and alcohol dependence;
- assessment and management of drug dependence and pregnancy;
- management of secondary complications of drug use.

It is essential to remember that detoxification is only the first step in the treatment process and without ongoing counselling and support relapse is high. Statistics for in-patient services give a rate of success of between 35 and 81% (Strang *et al.* 1997), with those for out-patients varying between 16 and 70% (Akhurst 1999; Day 2005). It is important to plan detoxification on occasion for medical reasons. In this case detoxification will take place as part of an emergency admission to either an acute medical bed or a psychiatric bed. Detoxification should take place when the client feels ready to manage the process. Symptoms after the last dose of opiate will begin within a few hours and can last for up to 5 days. During detoxification the client will need support and to be able to form a therapeutic relationship with his or her counsellor to talk about the issues. According to Mynors-Wallis *et al.* (2002) the symptoms of opiate withdrawal include:

- sweating
- yawning
- change in temperature (hot/cold)
- abdominal cramps
- anorexia
- nausea and/or vomiting
- aches and pains
- goose flesh
- dilated pupils
- tachycardia
- hypertension
- anxiety
- depression

Residential rehabilitation

Residential rehabilitation fits into tier 4 of the models of care (National Treatment Agency for Substance Misuse 2002). Most residential programmes require clients to be drug free before they enter the programme. Programmes will run for between 6 weeks and 12 months depending on client need. There are a limited number of residential rehabilitation centres that will take clients with substance misuse and mental health issues. Residential rehabilitation aims to maintain abstinence and provide communal living based on a group counselling approach. It can include employment experience, training and education. Residential rehabilitation will also provide ongoing support following discharge and assist with housing and resettlement (Gossop 2006).

Structured day services

Structured day services provide clients with formalised group work, including discussion related to substances. It will include discussion on relapse prevention and cravings, motivational interviewing and offer an element of support. It can be from a few sessions to several weeks.

Cognitive behavioural therapy

Cognitive behavioural therapy has been identified as providing good short-term outcomes for substance users (Department of Health 2006). It can be provided on an individual or a group basis. Didactic in approach, the therapist works on a structured approach to treatment. It uses both cognitive and environmental methods to allow clients to develop skills to manage their addiction. Cognitive behavioural therapy encourages clients to rehearse coping skills for the future.

Relapse prevention

Relapse prevention is essential to enable clients to understand the triggers that lead to relapse and to equip them with the skills to reduce their substance misuse or to remain abstinent. It is useful to apply the technique to high-risk situations and to practise for relapse as part of the treatment process. Marlatt and Gordon (1985) distinguish between the study of the relapse process and the clinical interventions that are intended to modify it. When looking at strategies to aid relapse prevention, relapse should be seen as a process in its own right and should be part of the after-care plan. Relapse prevention is based on both social and cognitive psychology and incorporates models of relapse along with behavioural and cognitive strategies. Relapse refers to a breakdown or failure in a person's attempt to maintain change in any set of behaviours. Relapse rates in any use of substance after a period of abstinence are notoriously high (Gossop 2006). Relapse needs to be viewed as part of the process of chronic illness and sometimes one just has to accept relapse and move on. Indeed, some clients may opt for controlled or occasional use of substances.

The relapse prevention process really begins before the first post-treatment session. It should include assessment of the home environment, the social environment, the person's response to situations, how you are going to work together, and the person's motivation to change (Parks and Marlatt 2000). A period of abstinence from substances will result in the client feeling confident (usually around 6 months free of substances). To maintain awareness that relapse is a real possibility the client should be prepared for self-help groups or the 12 Step Model (alcoholism.about.com 2007). The 12 Step Model is based on the Minnesota approach developed on the principles of Alcoholics Anonymous. It views addiction as a disease and works towards recovery but not cure. The programme offers support for drug/alcohol users involving group support, lectures and one-to-one counselling. It follows 12 principles: honesty, faith, surrender, soul searching, integrity, acceptance, humility, willingness, forgiveness, maintenance, making contact and service. It works with individuals who want to change their life as well as their addiction.

Change will only occur if there are other goals and as part of an overall care plan. Based on the client it could include:

- supported employment;
- leisure activities;
- normative relationships;
- social skills training;
- challenging self-defeating cognitions;
- expressing negative feelings.

Other things that can assist in the change process are:

- where the patient defines the problem;
- if there is the formation of a therapeutic alliance that avoids power struggles;
- where the successes of the patient are highlighted;
- where the patient's view of self is examined.

On occasions there will be relapses and these can be to do with:

- ineffective coping response;
- decreased self-efficacy;
- abstinence violation;
- negative emotional states (anger, anxiety, depression, boredom, frustration).

Cravings and urges can also be a problem in relation to relapse. Part of understanding relapse is to do with understanding cravings and the client learning to control and manage the cravings. Cravings come from physiological states. Cravings can be triggered by environmental stimuli, for example visiting a place where a client previously obtained drugs or going to a friend's house where he/she would normally drink. Relapse can also be triggered by an urge to respond to a sudden impulse for the substance. Cravings can be a subjective desire to experience the effects of the drug/alcohol. This can incorporate a desire for immediate gratification, as a reaction to direct or indirect social pressure. It can also be based on habit. High-risk situations can be any situation or condition that poses a threat to the individual's sense of self-efficacy and may include:

- negative emotional states;
- interpersonal conflict;
- social pressure;
- coping responses;
- awareness.

Relapse prevention therapy promotes the client's ability to understand relapse as a process and enables the client to identify and cope effectively with high-risk situations. The methodology teaches how to cope with urges and cravings and be able to implement damage control procedures during a lapse to minimise its negative consequences. It enables the client to stay engaged in treatment even after a relapse and allows the client to learn how to create a more balanced lifestyle. When dealing with high-risk situations it teaches understanding of the following:

- coping skills;
- outcome expectancies;
- abstinence violation effect;
- lifestyle imbalances;
- urges;
- cravings;
- social situations.

Issues that can affect the client's ability to maintain abstinence will include the following:

- High-risk situations
  – for example: decreased self-efficacy, rule violation, dissonance conflict (individual beliefs) and lifestyle imbalance.
- Insight/awareness
  – for example: coping skills, self image, risk situations or future dangers, early warning signs, planning the week ahead and alternative routes.
- Assessment
  – for example: focus on behaviour, look at control variables, self-monitoring diaries, including high-risk situations, number of units taken each day and social situations.
- The Plan
  – for example: framework for proactive interventions, concrete all-or-nothing plans, cognitive/behavioural models, assessment, insight/awareness, skills training, cognitive strategies and lifestyle interventions.
- Cognitive strategies
  – for example: cognitive restructuring – change patterns of thinking, relapse rehearsal – teaching client coping strategies and rehearsing them, coping imagery – talk about issues, visualise process, and allow craving to wash over client.
- Problem solving
  – for example: coping mechanisms, increased self-efficacy or mastery over behaviour, eliminating myths, anticipating relapse, knowing the relapse process and exploring the journey.
- Skill training
  – for example: relaxation training, assertiveness training, cue exposure, cravings, aromatherapy, reflexology, massage, auricular puncture.
- Lifestyle interventions
  – for example: lifestyle balance – ways of changing lifestyle, substitute indulgences – change craving to a reward, positive addictions – not an immediate positive outcome, and stimulus control techniques – minimise exposure to stimuli.

- Managing relapse
  - for example: focus on halting relapse; provide a non-judgemental approach; evaluate situation for clues; see it as part of journey; use cognitive structure and reframing to look at perceptions – not to see it as a failure but as the need for more planning and as a key learning opportunity; reframe warning signals; examine triggers, environment, associates, situation, events leading to relapse, future steps.
- Case studies
  - for example: change is a slow process, relapse is not failure, associate with own issues, and success can only be measured based on client need.
- Remembering
  - for example: accept that such feelings are natural, convert the feelings into positive action, let go client's choice, do not take it home with you, learn from it, see other clients who are doing well, and relapse is as educational as sobriety.

Risk reduction

Risk reduction is the proactive involvement of specialist drug/alcohol staff as soon as substance misuse is identified. Furthermore the prevention and management of violence training must include the specific issues associated with drug/alcohol use. It may be useful to work with the local police on managing substance misuse. It is important to have agreed policies and procedures in place, that a full risk assessment is completed, and that staff working within all areas of mental health and forensic services are trained in substance misuse.

Harm minimisation

Harm reduction has to be considered a large part of health promotion that is a fundamental part of substance misuse services. There has been much debate about harm reduction techniques and their relevance to services when working with clients who also have mental health issues. For some individuals it is a way to engage in services, as the thought of being completely abstinent appears to be an unrealistic goal, but reduction or minimisation of harm is a goal within reach. Harm minimisation advice needs to be given as part of a whole system of care aimed at improving the client's outcomes and enabling the client to make choices towards a better prognosis.

Harm reduction is based on reducing or stopping injecting. It aims to teach safer injecting techniques, to reduce or stop the sharing of equipment, to teach cleaning of equipment and, if sharing, cleaning equipment between sharing. It also involves discussion and help in accessing testing and counselling for:

- HIV/AIDS;
- hepatitis B and C;
- hepatitis B vaccination programmes;
- safer sex.

   Needle exchange services are run by both drug teams and chemists, who can provide users with needles, syringes, condoms, citric acid and sharps bins to provide protection to clients and the general public with safe disposal of sharps. Needle exchange is not available in prisons or forensic services.

Risk management in mental health settings

Risk assessment

Any risk assessment should include risk to self which is related to drug/ alcohol use, mental health symptoms, self-harm and also risk to others. This should also include any past history of violence, drugs/alcohol and mental health (Department of Health 2001b). Violence and risk assessment have become a key issue as services move to becoming community based. Swartz *et al.* (1998) note that clients who have non-compliance with medication, mental health issues, low levels of insight into mental health issues and who use substances are associated with serious violent incidents in the community. Any concerns for risk to children should also follow local child protection policies. There is no evidence to suggest that children of drug/ alcohol users are at greater risk, but a full risk assessment is needed. The Appelbaum *et al.* (2000) study of violence and delusions concluded that in terms of risk assessment, delusions did not relate to violent behaviour but did relate to mislabelling when clients reported delusions. There are no clear indicators to prevent drug use, but there are indicators to demonstrate risk factors and these include those reported in Box 7.2.

Risk management

Risk assessment and management should offer harm minimisation advice that includes discussion on drug overdose and risks that occur following periods of abstinence.

   Assessment is a complex procedure which takes place over a period of time. An initial assessment and history will be taken, but an ultimate decision regarding appropriate treatment may take longer if the person has a mental issue that is related to substance misuse. It is essential to involve both clients and carers in the process and in the development and

Box 7.2   Risk factors to drug use (Robinson 1999).

- Homelessness
- Social exclusion
- Self-harm
- Suicide
- Abuse
- Overdose
- Crime related to obtaining drugs/alcohol
- Risk to the client related to drug-using equipment, e.g. injuries as a result of inappropriate disposal of needles and syringes, cans, pipes, etc.
- Blood-borne infections due to sharing equipment, e.g. hepatitis, HIV
- Risk of overdose – accidental overdose on illicit substances, risk of not being able to obtain help
- Risk to others – violence can result following drug use
- Risk from others who become violent due to drug use
- Relapse and return to drug/alcohol use following a period of abstinence may lead to overdose
- Risk associated with an illegal activity
- Issues related to child care
- Indicators of relapse
- Factors known to increase risk
- Psychiatric diagnosis
- Non-compliance with medication
- Fire
- Absconsion
- Accommodation
- Use of weapons
- Impulsive behaviour
- Risks to children
- Exploitation by others
- Lack of meaningful occupation

review of their care plan. It is also essential to provide support for carers.

Discussion needs to take place regarding types and supply of drugs as the purity of drugs will depend on supply and some may be more pure than others. This may result in overdose if a client is not used to an increased purity level. In the management of risk it is important to discuss high-risk behaviours, e.g. sharing equipment, including needles, syringes, spoons and drugs, and unsafe sexual practices.

When managing risk it is fundamental to the process to ensure a plan is in place to reduce the risk of substance misuse relapse and promote adherence to the current treatment plan. Risk factors for dual diagnosis in studies of twins (Kendler *et al.* 2003) demonstrated that the environment has an effect on choice of substance used but not where the person would become dependent. The risk factor in dual diagnosis for relapse is higher when combined with a personality disorder (Abdulrahim 2001). Clinicians need to ensure a clear plan is in place that incorporates both mental health issues and substance misuse. Within this plan there needs to be incorporated what measures would be implemented should the client become non-compliant with medication or disengage with services. A client with a primary mental health diagnosis of psychosis and substance misuse is more likely to have poor conformity to medication and engagement.

Hawkins *et al.* (1992) recognise that short-term abstinence is easier to achieve than long-term abstinence, and support and long-term relapse prevention need to be considered. Risk management of substance misuse goes hand in hand with criminal laws because it is an illegal activity and deliberation needs to be given to this when managing the situation. In recent years the availability and cost of drugs and alcohol has reduced. This has led to an increase in drug and alcohol use. It is not the healthcare professionals' role to police drugs and alcohol in hospital, but it is their role to ensure that the issues are dealt with in line with current hospital policy and in liaison with the police.

Christie *et al.* (1988) demonstrated an increased risk of drug abuse or dependence in conjunction with a major depressive episode. It is also worth considering the reaction to stress in vulnerable individuals when working with relapse prevention as exposure to stress can increase drug use and also the associations with cravings and relapse (Sinha 2001). It is important to record the context of the risk and share information as agreed under employers' protocols. Most workers do not consider risk to themselves when working with known substance users (Wright *et al.* 2006).

Rosenberg *et al.* (1998) developed the Dartmouth Assessment of Lifestyle Instrument (DALI) to enable staff to screen for drug or alcohol use alongside mental health assessment. It demonstrates the need to assess mental health and substance use together for a comprehensive assessment. When managing risk it is important to consider the following:

- choice of care co-ordinator based on clinical need, worker from either drug or community mental health team;
- crisis plan;
- service user and carer comments;
- contingency plan;
- vulnerable adults meeting;
- child protection;
- referral to public protection panel;
- risk assessment meeting;
- cultural issues;
- whether screening takes place.

Risk assessment and management in forensic settings

Prisoners have a high incidence of substance misuse and mental health problems (Department of Health 2002b). As part of the Criminal Justice and Court Services Act (2001), drug testing is required at all stages of the criminal process. Drug Treatment and Testing Orders (DTTOs) were introduced to ensure offenders experiencing substance misuse have access to substance misuse services and mental health services.

Gunn (2000) identifies high levels of mental ill health in prisons and reports that 4–10% of prisoners on remand and 2–7% of sentenced prisoners present with a psychosis. Substance misuse is a considerable problem for both prisons and forensic settings. Hodgins and Muler-Isberner (2004) demonstrated that 77.8% of the forensic patients in his study had previously been admitted to a general psychiatric service and 24.3% of the general psychiatric patients had a criminal record. Both mental health and substance misuse exacerbate the role of substance misuse in youth offending, along with non-compliance to prescribed medication. This can lead to a risk of violence. Dual diagnosis is associated with an increased use of services and an increased possibility of becoming involved in offending behaviour.

As prisons have reached an all-time high for admissions, substance misuse and mental health have become a concern in terms of managing risk. Work streams currently taking place include health and offender partnerships, care services improvement partnership, health and social care criminal justice programmes, and prison health – all aimed at working with healthcare professionals to offer a comprehensive service including risk assessment and management for service users with offending behaviour. O'Grady (2001) recognises there is a link between substance misuse, mental health and violence.

In forensic settings, for risk assessment the following need to be considered:

- all the above factors for mental health services users;
- are all clients routinely assessed for substance misuse?
- who is likely to be vulnerable;
- victims of crime;
- perpetrators of crime;
- availability of specialist addiction services;
- victims of abuse;
- how will follow-up be completed for clients admitted from non-catchment areas?
- women are more likely to report substance misuse.

One of the key issues for forensic settings is that the development of services has been different across the country and more information is

Box 7.3   Case study 2: Jon

Jon is a 40-year-old Afro Caribbean male. Jon has a history of using cannabis (skunk and resin), heroin, amphetamines and alcohol. He still uses cannabis, heroin and alcohol. Jon has in the past used various methods including injecting, ingestion, smoking, snorting and chasing.

Jon has a diagnosis of borderline personality disorder with psychotic features and was previously diagnosed with paranoid schizophrenia. He has a long history of childhood sexual abuse. Jon has recently come out of prison following an 8-year sentence for unlawful sexual intercourse, and has numerous previous prison sentences for assault, theft and aggravated assault. He has been made homeless on a number of occasions and worked as a rent boy in the past. Jon has never been in touch with mental health services and has received a diagnosis via the prison service. He is currently on the sex offender's register and is supervised by a probation officer. He is housed on a housing estate and is in debt. He maintains debts by running errands for dealers. Jon currently has memory deficits when drinking alcohol.

He has difficulty in engaging with services. Information sharing with probation service is problematic.

Jon is currently receiving care via the following services:

- probation;
- dual diagnosis nurse to talk about harm minimisation and work on relapse prevention.

The following risk factors can be identified:

- risk of violence from dealers;
- risk of relapse to crime;
- risk from drug and alcohol relapse;
- risk to children as Jon is on sex offenders register;
- non-compliance with medication;
- previous history of being homeless.

Jon finds it difficult to engage in services and trust people; having spent most of his life in custodial care, he verbalises compliance and fails to attend appointments. He does not want to share issues regarding abuse with probation worker.

Engagement is the key to assisting Jon. The dual diagnosis nurse works weekly on relapse prevention and sexual abuse issues. The nurse encourages him to share information with probation, works in line with trust policies for sharing of information and is clear with the client regarding child protection issues. The key to maintaining Jon in services is confidentiality and prescribing for his heroin use. Social links need to be maintained including ensuring he maintains his accommodation through debt management. Because of his previous forensic history it is essential that a full risk assessment is carried out by forensic services and a management plan is in place that includes risk to children.

---

required on admissions to forensic and to local psychiatric services (Coid *et al.* 2001). Case study 2 in Box 7.3 addresses issues of risk and how important it is that interactions between services take place in assessing that risk.

Conclusion

Dual diagnosis carries greater risks than most other areas of mental health because of the effect of substances on people's mental health and because of the lifestyle they may maintain to ensure their access to drugs or alcohol. This may include levels of violence, crime and contact with criminal justice systems. The key to ensuring individuals do not slip through the net is early detection and treatment. Full comprehensive assessments need to be in place that ask about every aspect of drug or alcohol use, as well as effective screening of urine or saliva on admission. Mental health symptoms can be masked by the use of drugs or alcohol and can also be exacerbated. Using substances should not rule out assessment, but if clearly intoxicated, assessment should be delayed but the individual should still be screened.

There need to be clear protocols related to risk assessment for this client group that are linked to clinical governance and government and trust policies and collaborative working between drug/alcohol teams and mental health services. This is currently being developed jointly by trusts and Drug Action Teams but can only be maintained by clinical teams. This client group needs clear policies that include substance misuse as an acceptable and treatable issue and over which they can freely discuss issues without fear of discharge. This does not mean acceptance of drug/alcohol use on wards but ensuring that clients have access to prescribing, detoxification and group work on admission. A clear indicator is the number of individuals who discharge themselves in order to continue their drug use because they cannot see any other solution.

Group work is the key to success with this client group as relapse is high and needs to be regarded as part of the process and not as a failure. With increasing acceptance in society that drug and alcohol use is part of the social norm even when not legal it is essential that healthcare professionals develop services to meet this need. It is essential that all healthcare professionals are trained in risk management and substance misuse to enable them to provide the appropriate level of care to individuals with a dual diagnosis. Dual diagnosis is not a specialist service because of the levels of drug/alcohol use and needs all staff to be aware of the issues. It is important to remember that for some individuals drugs/alcohol have maintained their mental health, and appropriate risk assessment and treatment need to be in place before detoxification to ensure appropriate care is provided.

References

Abdulrahim, D. (2001) *Substance Misuse and Mental Health Co-Morbidity (Dual Diagnosis)*. Health Advisory Service, London.

Akhurst, J.S. (1999) The use of lofexidine by drug dependency units in the United Kingdom. *European Addiction Research*, **5**(1), 43–49.

alcoholism.about.com (2007) *The Twelve Steps: A Guide Toward an Entire New Way of Life*. Available at http://alcoholism.about.com/cs/info/a/aa981021.htm (accessed 29 October 2007).

Alexander, M.J. & Haugland, G. (2000) *Integrating Services for Co-Occurring Disorders: Final Report Prepared for the New York State Conference of Local Mental Hygiene Directors*. Center for the Study of Issues in Public Mental Health, Orangeburg, New York.

Appelbaum, P.S., Robbins, P.C. & Monahan, J. (2000) Violence and delusions: data from the MacArthur violence risk assessment study. *American Journal of Psychiatry*, **157**, 566–572.

Appleby, L., Shaw, J. & Amos, T., *et al.* (1999) *Safer Services. Report of the National Confidential Inquiry into Suicide and Homicide by People with Mental Illness*. Department of Health, London.

Ashton, C.H. (2006) *Benzodiazepines: Problems and Solutions*. All-Party Action Group on Tranquilliser Addiction, House of Commons, London, 7 November. Available at http://www.benzo.org.uk/hoc711.htm (accessed 22 October 2007).

Bennetto, J. (2006) Drug nation. *The Independent*, 13 September, pp. 1–2.

Chick, J. & Cantwell, R. (1994) Aetiology of alcohol misuse. *British Journal of Addiction*, **82**, 147–157.

Christie, K.A., Burke, J.D., Regier, D.A., Rae, D.S., Boyd, J.H. & Locke, B.Z. (1988) Epidemiologic evidence for early onset of mental disorders and high risk of drug abuse in young adults. *American Journal of Psychiatry*, **145**, 971–975

Coid, J., Kahtan, N., Gault, S., Cook, A. & Jarman, B. (2001) Medium secure forensic psychiatry services: comparison of seven English health regions. *British Journal of Psychiatry*, **178**, 55–61.

Day, E. (2005) *Opiate Detoxification in an In-Patient Setting*. National Treatment Agency for Substance Misuse, London.

Department of Health (1990) *Caring for People: The Care Programme Approach for People with a Mental Illness Referred to the Specialist Psychiatric Services*. Department of Health, London.

Department of Health (1996) *Building Bridges: A Guide to Arrangements for Inter-Agency Working for the Care and Protection of Severely Mentally Ill People*. Department of Health, London.

Department of Health (1998) *Tackling Drugs Together to Build a Better Britain*. Department of Health, London.

Department of Health (1999) *Mental Health National Service Framework: Modern Standards and Service Models.* Department of Health, London.

Department of Health (2000) *The NHS Plan: A Plan for Investment: A Plan for Reform.* Department of Health, London.

Department of Health (2001a) *The Essence of Care: Patient-Focused Benchmarking for Health Care Practitioners.* Department of Health, London.

Department of Health (2001b) *Safety First: Five-Year Report of the National Confidential Inquiry into Suicide and Homicide by People with Mental Illness.* Department of Health, London.

Department of Health (2002a) *Developing an Integrated Model of Care for Substance Abuse Treatment.* Department of Health, London.

Department of Health (2002b) *Dual Diagnosis Good Practice Guide.* Department of Health, London.

Department of Health (2004) *The National Service Framework for Mental Health – Five Years On.* Department of Health, London.

Department of Health (2005) *Delivering Race Equality in Mental Health Care: An Action Plan for Reform Inside and Outside Services and the Government's Response to the Independent Inquiry into the Death of David Bennett.* Department of Health, London.

Department of Health (2006) *Dual Diagnosis in Mental Health Inpatient and Day Hospital Settings.* Department of Health, London.

Drake, R.E., Osher, F.C. & Wallach, M.A. (1989) Alcohol use and abuse in schizophrenia: a prospective community study. *Journal of Nervous and Mental Disease*, **177**, 408–414.

Drake, R.E., Mercer-McFannen, C., Mueser, K.T., McHugo, G.J. & Bond, G.R. (1998) A review of integrated mental health and substance abuse treatment for people with dual disorders. *Schizophrenia Bulletin*, **24**(4), 589–608.

Eliany, M. & Rush, B. (1992) *The Effectiveness of Prevention and Treatment Programs for Alcohol and Other Drug Problems: A Review of Evaluation Studies* (unpublished report). Health and Welfare Canada, Ottawa.

Ewing, J.A. (1984) Detecting alcoholism: the CAGE questionnaire. *Journal of American Medical Association*, **252**, 1905–1907.

Gavin, D.R., Ross, H.E. & Skinner, H.A. (1989) Diagnostic validity of the Drug Abuse Screening Test (DAST) in the assessment of DSM-III drug disorders. *British Journal of Addiction*, **84**(3), 301–307

Gelder, M., Mayou, R. & Cowen, P. (2001) *Shorter Oxford Textbook of Psychiatry.* Oxford University Press, Oxford.

Gossop, M. (2006) *Treating Drug Misuse Problems: Evidence of Effectiveness.* National Treatment Agency for Substance Misuse, London. Available at http://www.nta.nhs.uk/publications/documents/nta_treat_drug_misuse_evidence_effectiveness_2006_rb5.pdf (accessed 29 October 2007).

Gunn, J. (2000) Future directions for treatment in forensic psychiatry. *British Journal of Psychiatry*, **176**, 332–338.

Hawkins, J.D., Catalano, R.F. & Miller, J.Y. (1992) Risk and protective factors for alcohol and other drug problems in adolescence and early childhood. *Psychological Bulletin*, **112**(1), 64–105.

Health Services and Utilization and Research Council (2001) *Getting Started with Integrated Care Pathways*. Available at http://www.hqc.sk.ca/download. jsp?iPh/ADwc2TovRhvh6/qyPDBIzBf0QfLQkUwK4QBZaJs1HJ7Eha+/ uA= = (accessed 29 October 2007).

Hodgins, S. & Muler-Isberner, R. (2004) Preventing crime by people with schizophrenic disorders: the role of psychiatric services. *British Journal of Psychiatry*, **185**, 245–250.

Hughes, L. (2006) *Closing the Gap: A Capability Framework for Working Effectively with People with Combined Mental Health and Substance Use Problems (Dual Diagnosis)*. Centre for Clinical and Academic Workforce Innovation, University of Lincoln.

Johns, A. (1997) Substance misuse: a primary risk and a major problem of comorbidity. *International Review of Psychiatry*, **9**(2–3), 233–245.

Kendler, K.S., Jacobson, K.C., Prescott, C.A. & Neale, M.C. (2003) Specificity of genetic and environmental factors for use and abuse/dependence of cannabis, cocaine, hallucinogens, sedatives, stimulants, and opiates in male twins. *American Journal of Psychiatry*, **160**, 687–695.

Marlatt, A. & Gordon, J. (1985) *Relapse Prevention Maintenance Strategies in the Treatment of Addictive Disorders*. Guildford Press, New York.

McHugo, G.J., Drake, R.E., Burton, H.L. & Ackerson, T.H. (1995) A scale for assessing the stage of substance abuse treatment in persons with severe mental illness. *Journal of Nervous and Mental Disease*, **183**(12), 762–767.

Miller, W.R. & Rollnick, W. (1998) *Motivational Interviewing: Preparing People to Change. Professional Training Videotape Series*. University of New Mexico, Albuquerque.

Miller, W.R. & Rollnick, S. (2002) *Motivational Interviewing: Preparing People for Change*, 2nd edn. Guilford Press, New York.

Mynors-Wallis, L., Moore, M., Maguire, J. & Hollingbery, T. (2002) *Shared Care in Mental Health*. Oxford University Press, Oxford.

National Treatment Agency for Substance Misuse (2002) *Models of Care for the Treatment of Drug Misusers: Promoting Quality, Efficiency and Effectiveness in Drug Misuse Treatment Services in England. Part 2: Full Reference Report*. National Treatment Agency for Substance Misuse, London.

National Treatment Agency for Substance Misuse (2004) *Drugs and Alcohol in the Workplace*. National Treatment Agency for Substance Misuse, London. Available at www.nta.nhs.uk/publications/documents/nta_drugs_and_ alcohol_in_the_workplace_2004_ddsp3.pdf (accessed 10 December 2007).

National Treatment Agency for Substance Misuse (2007a) *New National Statistics Reveal More Drug Users in Treatment.* National media release: 18 October 2007. Available at http://www.nta.nhs.uk/media/media_releases /2007_media_releases/new_national_statistics_reveal_more_drug_users_ in_treatment_media_release_181007.aspx (accessed 22 October 2007).

National Treatment Agency for Substance Misuse (2007b) *New Funding Distribution Formula for Drug Treatment in England.* National media release: 29 January 2007. Available at http://www.nta.nhs.uk/media/media_ releases/2007_media_releases/new_funding_distribution_formula_ for_drug_treatment_in_england_290107.aspx (accessed 22 October 2007).

Office of National Statistics (1997) *Psychiatric Morbidity in Prisoners in England and Wales.* Office of National Statistics, London.

O'Grady, J. (2001) Commentary. *Advances in Psychiatric Treatment*, **7**, 196–197.

Parks, G.A. & Marlatt, G.A. (2000) Relapse prevention therapy: a cognitive behavioural approach. *The National Psychologist*, **9**(5). Available at http:// nationalpsychologist.com/articles/art_v9n5_3.htm (accessed 29 October 2007).

Phillips, P. (2000) Substance misuse, offending and mental illness: a review. *Journal of Psychiatric and Mental Health Nursing*, **7**(6), 483–489.

Prins, H. (2005) *Offenders, Deviants or Patients?* 3rd edn. Routledge, Taylor and Francis, London.

Prochaska, J.O. & DiClemente, C.C. (1983) Stages and processes of self-change of smoking: toward an integrative model of change. *Journal of Consulting and Clinical Psychology*, **51**, 390–395.

Raistrick, D.S., Bradshaw, J., Tober, G., Weiner, J., Allison, J. & Healey, C. (1994) Development of the Leeds Dependence Questionnaire. *Addiction*, **89**, 563–572.

Robinson, P. (1999) *Forbidden Drugs: Understanding Drugs and Why People Take Them*, 2nd edn. Oxford University Press, Oxford.

Rosenberg, S.D., Drake, R.E., Wolford, G.L., *et al.* (1998) Dartmouth Assessment of Lifestyle Instrument (DALI): a substance use disorder screen for people with severe mental illness. *American Journal of Psychiatry*, **155**, 232–238.

Selzer, M.L. (1971) The Michigan Alcohol Screening Test (MAST). The quest for a new diagnostic instrument. *American Journal of Psychiatry*, **127**, 1653–1658

Sinha, R. (2001) How does stress increase risk of drug abuse and relapse? *Psychopharmacology*, **158**(4), 343–359.

Strang, J., Marks, I., Dawe, S., Powell, J., Gossop, M., Richards, D. & Gray, J. (1997) Type of hospital setting and treatment outcome with heroin addicts. *British Journal of Psychiatry*, **171**, 335–339.

Swartz, M.S., Swanson, J.W., Hiday, A.A., Borum, R., Wagner, H.R. & Burns, B.J. (1998) Violence and severe mental illness: the effects of substance abuse and non-adherence to medication. *American Journal of Psychiatry*, **155**, 226–231.

Wright, C., Kramer, E.D., Zalman, M.A., Smith, M.Y. & Haddox, J.D. (2006) Risk identification, risk assessment, and risk management of abusable drug formulations. *Drug and Alcohol Dependence*, **83**(Supplement 1), S68–S76.

Chapter 8

Conclusions

Alyson M. Kettles and Phil Woods

Introduction

The content of this book has shown that risk assessment in mental health nursing is not a single, static entity, but a complex issue involving many aspects of the person being assessed and the contribution of other factors such as situational ones. There has been an evolving history for the last 30 years which shows that mental health nurses have been involved in using risk assessments and in managing the care of patients deemed to be at any level of risk. However, recently, mental health nurses have been much more proactively involved in the development of risk assessment scales (Almvik *et al.* 2000; Almvik and Woods 2003; Ross *et al.* 2008; Woods 2008) and in the development of clinical management approaches (Doyle 2000; Woods and Kettles 2007). This shows the continuing trend for nurses to be directly involved in the development of care and in ensuring patient and public safety through risk assessment and management processes.

Not only has there been a history of nursing involvement in risk assessment, but this development has to be set against the policy and legislative backdrop that has enabled it. Policy and legislation have moved (relatively) quickly to make major changes in the four countries that make up the United Kingdom. Scotland has led the way with the implementation of the European Human Rights legislation through both mental health law and the policy surrounding it, including the setting up of the Risk Management Authority. Policy across the globe is changing towards a much more rights and recovery based focus and this means fundamental changes in the ways in which we work as nurses, except in one respect.

Nursing has always meant that we engage with people, that we walk with them through their journey and that we communicate at all stages of care. This has not and will not change regardless of changes to legislation, policy, education and professional development. Risk assessment is not just a tool of the trade to be used in a mechanical fashion. Risk assessment is about getting to know the person in the way that nurses have always done and working with them to manage or alleviate any risks. Risk assessment may be more systematic than we were used to fifty or a hundred years ago, but, in essence, it remains about knowing the person and the likelihood of behaviours occurring, then preventing or dealing appropriately with those behaviours. Engagement is based on the premise that the relationship enables safe, appropriate and therapeutic care to be carried out with patients on their journey, through their lives or through our particular parts of the service or both. We may have had some 'notion' of risk 50 years ago, but it was often based on the nurse's professional judgement or on intuition.

Today, we recognise that the nurse's professional judgement needs to be based on as much available information as possible and that nurses do not act in isolation but work very much as part of a team. Professional judgement is now questioned during legal processes, such as Fatal Accident Inquiries (FAIs). Moreover, without having as much knowledge as possible about the person and without having something concrete to go on, administering care that is based on intuition or solely on professional judgement is no longer acceptable.

Key messages

Depth, breadth and complexity

What has been seen throughout this book are the ways in which nurses are moving towards a much deeper understanding of assessment processes and tools in clinical practice with some of the most difficult client groups in mental health. Forensic mental health nursing has led the way forward through the risk assessment maze over the last 30 years or more, but mental health nursing in a more general sense is beginning to catch up with instruments designed for specific client groups to help to make clinical care as appropriate as it can be. In some respects this use in clinical practice is the missing link from the last 30 years, but this is beginning to change.

Initially, risk assessment tools were designed for research purposes, whereas today risk assessment tools are being designed with clinical utility in mind (Almvik *et al.* 2000; Almvik and Woods 2003; Ross *et al.* 2008; Woods 2008). One example is the BEST Index (Reed and Woods 2000) which was developed with the aim of giving a picture of clinical change over time, rather than previous actuarial scales that relied heavily on historical information giving only a one-off picture at a specific point in time. Another similar example would be the START (Webster *et al.* 2004). Many of these newer instruments have been designed with the intention of use with a range of different patient groups and are being utilised by mental health nurses in their everyday practice both in forensic and mainstream mental health settings.

What this book has also shown is that nurses can and do, with the appropriate training, assess the person's risk status just as ably as any other health professional. You should not be afraid to ask to be trained, to attend risk assessment information and training sessions, or to ask your manager for the funding to enable you to become fully educated in risk assessment and management.

'*Risk is a risky business*' (Prins 2002) is a well-known saying and one that emphasises the inexact nature of risk. Because we cannot be one hundred percent sure that our risk assessment is correct, we need to have conducted that risk assessment to the best of our ability. It needs to be carried out in such a way that people trust the process. All parties involved need to be certain that they have done the best they can for the patient, for the staff and other patients and carers, as well as for public safety. Rigorous assessment which accurately reflects the situation cannot be substituted with guesses, intuition or professional judgement. If you are charged with conducting a risk assessment, this information may be used not only to decide on the best way forward for a patient, but also in legal proceedings, and it may be used by a risk management authority to base decisions and actions on. Risk assessment is not only a risky business, it is also a serious business with long-term consequences for everyone involved.

Another point that this book has illustrated is the many facets of risk assessment that have to be taken into consideration. Risk assessment is not a quick and easy thing to do. It is not just about asking a few questions from a short screening tool, although that may be the start of the process. Risk assessment in mental health nursing is an ongoing process that has to be formally revisited on a regular basis and which needs to be carried out on a less formal basis continually. The process is a lengthy one with many questions, with observation and engagement as its fundamental relational method and with many particular points to be noted.

Increasing complexity is another characteristic of risk assessment in mental health nursing. Risk assessments are no longer one-page instruments but rather have evolved to become in-depth instruments that also give breadth to the presenting behaviours and status of the person coming into your service. These tools are developing in such a way as to fit with the current move towards values-based and recovery-focused care. As can be seen throughout the book, instruments are split into sections that deal with specific aspects of the potential risk that an individual might represent. These sections are assessments in themselves and present the opportunity for mental health nurses to conduct in-depth assessments, while the inclusion of several sections enables the breadth to be covered. It is possible, depending on the specific instrument and the way it has been designed, to use specific parts only. However, this would be for research purposes or for very specific clinical purposes. So, for example, although the whole BEST Index (Reed and Woods 2000) would be used for overall risk assessment at specified intervals, a nurse might wish to ascertain whether or not specific social skills were improving between complete risk assessments, and so might use the social skills component to check progress, or if specific problems were suspected and confirmation was required. However, it should always be checked with the authors whether or not a tool can be used in this way.

Both the preceding points, about many facets and increasing complexity, bring us to the issue of assessment of multiple risk and the different areas in which multiple risk may exist for mental health patients and staff. Multiple risks do not just occur in forensic mental health settings. Patients can come into mental healthcare through any avenue and can bring with them many potential risks. For example, a General Practitioner (GP) referring a patient to a Community Psychiatric Nurse (CPN) may be worried about a patient's state of mind, due to the break-up of the relationship with a girlfriend and warn the CPN that the patient *'may have his father's service revolver'*. So multiple risks are already present in the CPN's mind, without even meeting the patient, and include the risk of violence to the girlfriend, risk of suicide or self-harm, risk to others and the ever-present possibility of risk of substance misuse due to a depressive state.

This is also where the integration of screening, risk assessment and risk management come together. The CPN may take a variety of actions in relation to this potentially serious situation, with safety in mind. For example, contacting the CPN Manager and taking advice about how to deal with the situation, contacting the police for back-up, telephoning the patient to arrange a meeting, driving past the patient's residence to see what is happening or if there is anything visible, checking with the GP what exactly the patient said, and going to any meeting with the patient with another CPN – all this without having met the patient yet and with a view to assessing the situation, as well as the patient, in terms of risk.

This situation actually happened to the first author, but it had a reasonably happy ending because the patient did not have access to any firearms and it was all just threats, but at the time neither the GP nor the CPN knew that. The integration of safety with risk assessment and management is essential and has to be conducted with sensitivity and care.

Reliable instruments, reliably used = patient benefit

As the first author (Woods) points out in Chapter 4, rigour, reliability and validity are essential when developing or using risk assessment instruments. This is an 'old' concept but nevertheless it remains a fundamental issue about the whole process of assessment. Without rigorous application of properly validated and reliable instruments, the whole process of risk assessment can be called into question and frequently if for any reason litigation occurs. Throughout this book it has been reiterated that the education and training of staff in the use of validated instruments is essential to enable accuracy, inter-rater reliability and the facilitation of clinical utility.

Kettles *et al.* (2003) have shown that 63% of staff in forensic units use locally developed risk assessments and 7% were, at that time, developing their own. It is not known what the situation is in general mental health and acute mental areas; however, this will change later this year with an evaluation of the Clinical Resource and Audit Group (CRAG) (2002) document and the decision-making processes associated with risk assessment related to observation of the acutely ill patients in Scotland through research by the first author and colleagues, and with a review of the situation in Saskatchewan, Canada, by the second author. If the situation is as bad in acute areas as it is in forensic areas then this situation needs to be very carefully addressed at national level. This lack of reliable instruments in use in forensic areas does not have to be the case, as the first author has shown (Chapter 4) that there are a number of instruments already in existence that are appropriate and which have clinical utility.

Part of the problem about staff using reliable instruments continues to be that there is reluctance by staff to use instruments developed elsewhere, which may help to account for the persistence by staff in reinventing the wheel. This attitude of *'we will only use what we develop'* is a waste of everybody's time and it can even be deemed to be negligent, in that not providing the best possible care available is to the detriment of the patient and others. Therapeutic care begins with mental health nurses applying validated risk assessment to the patient situation and then it continues with a comprehensive risk management process and plan which encompasses the range of nursing and other interventions whilst incorporating recovery and values based care.

The future of risk assessment

Clearly there has been a developmental history of risk assessment and management in the last 30 years. This history has been characterised by:

- the search for predictive ability;
- validated instruments;
- increasing complexity;
- multidisciplinary involvement;
- process management;
- evolution of risk management authorities;
- the development of positive risk-taking as a therapeutic intervention;

- response to litigation;
- staff education.

However, given that this whole field began as a discussion of the meaning of 'dangerousness' we have come a very long way in a short time. So what of the future? Where are we heading? There are several points related to the future development of risk assessment.

First, mental health nurses are ideally placed to continue to develop specific therapeutic interventions related to the risk management process. We have seen the specific development of therapeutic and management interventions, such as positive risk taking (Morgan and Wetherell 2004) and flexible observation (Kettles and Paterson 2007), and there is little doubt that nurses will continue to develop interventions to meet patients' needs. As we become increasingly sophisticated in our knowledge and abilities in this field we will seek new ways to help patients and to manage the process.

Second, policy development will continue, but there are particular issues about policy that are not being addressed at the moment. For example, the first set of policy guidelines have been published for the prison service in England (Department of Health and HM Prison Service 2006) but not in Scotland. Also, two sets of guidelines have been published in Scotland (CRAG/SCOTMEG (Working Group on Mental Illness) 1995 and CRAG 2002), but there are no current plans to update these. So we have disparity between countries in the United Kingdom about the publication of guidelines and no set review dates for those that have been published. In addition to this there have been no 'official' reviews or evaluations of these published guidelines. All these issues need to be addressed as a matter of urgency if there is to be consistent and appropriate care given to patients at risk. The first and most important issue is the setting of regular review dates for policy and guideline development; this should be carried out every 2–4 years as more work is done to take risk assessment and associated intervention forward.

Third, getting staff to accept the need for validated instruments and training those staff in their use is, in itself, an enormous challenge. There needs to be a concerted effort in future in educating and training mental health nurses to use instruments properly. Let's stop wasting all this effort on re-inventing the wheel. This work needs to be led by the official nurses' bodies, such as the Nurses and Midwives Council in the UK and NHS Education for Scotland. It is no use individuals being trained and then finding themselves unable to use their training because no-one else in their area is doing it. Also, currently in the Risk Management Authority in Scotland there are only two qualified risk assessors (one psychiatrist and one psychologist), who cover the whole of Scotland because people, who may be eligible, are unwilling to put themselves through the rigorous selection process to become accredited risk assessors. This is a major problem that needs to be worked on for the future and the starting place is to train people from the beginning, not as some kind of afterthought. New degrees, such as the BSc (Hons) in Professional Practice (Violence Reduction) at the University of Glamorgan (http://www.glam.ac.uk/coursedetails/685/688), aim to redress this balance somewhat, but even they do not qualify the student in the specific use of risk assessment instruments but only include 'an overview' of the instruments themselves.

Fourth, continuing development of both clinical and predictive risk assessment tools is essential. As this book has shown there is a clear way forward for the structured clinical judgement approach and more research is required here to improve the issue.

Risk assessment research

Mental health nurse researchers face an uphill battle, with few permanent jobs, increasing competition for available funding and less money available for training and education to become qualified researchers. In addition to all this, they face the problems of research into risk assessment. Competition comes particularly from the psychologists in the field, but mental health nurse researchers can find both mainstream and niche markets available into risk assessment research.

For example, in mainstream research large-scale funding can be applied for in both developmental and validation research into the utility of new and existing instruments. Also, there are many areas of mainstream research that either have not been addressed or have only had initial and/or pilot research conducted, for example the relationship between risk assessment and specific interventions such as observation or engagement. There are also niche markets that enable staff to enter the field, such as planning audits which then move on into research. For example, local audits of risk assessment processes can reveal areas that lend themselves to research, such as information provision to patients, management of incidents, complaints procedures and the knowledge, attitudes and training of staff to use specific instruments.

One of the single biggest problems with nursing research in the field of risk assessment is that many nurses are uncomfortable working with numbers. Validated and reliable risk assessment instruments require staff who can work with quantitative data and many nurses in mental health only feel comfortable working with qualitative methods of research. This is a particular barrier in nursing (not just mental health nursing) and one that needs to be overcome through nursing degree courses demanding the same professional levels of entry as any other profession. Only then will this problem with numeracy be overcome. Risk assessment research demands an ability to use numbers appropriately to be able to develop and to validate instruments. However, as has been noted earlier, it is not the ability to use numbers that is the most important issue in research but the manner and approach that is used by the researcher in pursuit of the knowledge about risk assessment.

A variety of approaches to risk assessment

Risk assessment has been addressed in a variety of ways within this book. Through these approaches a number of themes have been identified. For example, John Cordall in Chapter 2 provided us with a very thought-provoking chapter that aimed to give some insight into the concepts surrounding the whole issue of risk assessment and management. He reminded us that the history of risk assessment is founded on risk assessment failures and that risk assessments remain fallible. Fallibility is the issue that we aim to minimise as much as is possible. Primarily throughout the book the nurse–patient relationship has been identified as the single most important issue to prevent failure and to enable in-depth assessments to be conducted.

Kettles and Woods in Chapter 3 discussed the ideas around risk and defined terms for the purposes of this book. They also illustrated some of the newer forms of risk assessment that are emerging and how they are used to help mental health professionals to assess risk. The idea that risk assessment is a moveable feast was introduced here and the chapter showed that risk assessment is evolutionary with ongoing development.

Woods and Kettles gave a sound explication of the need for proper instrumentation in Chapter 4. They then went on to describe several instruments that are available for mental health nurses to use without having to develop local tools. These are good examples of the types of instruments that nurses can and do use. The issues of screening versus in-depth assessment were discussed and each shown to have an appropriate place in the process of risk assessment.

Woods in Chapter 5 showed that risk to others is not as straightforward as the media would have us believe. Emphasis on the skills of the mental health nurse shows that nurses are capable and have the skills to be able to use instruments to the benefit of others as well as the patient. Woods clearly showed the need for in-depth assessment and the need to be able to conduct it properly.

In Chapter 6 Lee Murray and Eve Upshall discussed risk to self through both suicidal behaviour and self-harming behaviour. The importance of the nurse–patient relationship was emphasised and reiterated. Integration of risk assessment in daily care was shown through the ADPIE system discussed in this chapter. Without appropriate integration into ward, clinical and daily functioning, risk assessment cannot work properly to the benefit of all.

Lois Dugmore in Chapter 7 enabled a greater understanding of the risk factors associated with substance misuse and the risk assessment and management tools and pathways that are in current use. Again the integration of risk assessment into care processes was shown in this chapter together with the risks that multiple use of substances can pose to both the individual and others.

All of this showed that there are a variety of possible approaches to care but that the fundamental issues remain the use of validated instruments and the sensitive application of them in clinical practice through integration of risk assessment into care and through appropriate development of the nurse–patient relationship.

Final note

It is hoped that some of the questions that were outlined in Chapter 1 of this book have been answered for the reader. No one book can answer all of these; however, it can help to pave the way forward for readers to look for answers to their own specific questions. It is clear from the content of this book that risk assessment and management in mental health nursing is developing at a pace and will undoubtedly continue to do so for the foreseeable future.

References

Almvik, R. & Woods, P. (2003) Short-term risk prediction: the Broset Violence Checklist. *Journal of Psychiatric and Mental Health Nursing*, **10**(2), 236–238.

Almvik, R., Woods, P. & Rasmussen, K. (2000) The Broset Violence Checklist (BVC): sensitivity, specificity and inter-rater reliability. *Journal of Interpersonal Violence*, **15**(12), 284–1296.

Clinical Resource and Audit Group (2002) *Engaging People: A Good Practice Statement*. Clinical Resource and Audit Group, Scottish Executive, Edinburgh.

CRAG/SCOTMEG (Working Group on Mental Illness) (1995) *Nursing Observation of Acutely Ill Psychiatric Patients in Hospital: A Good Practice Statement*. The Scottish Office, Edinburgh.

Department of Health and HM Prison Service (2006) *Mental Health Observation Including Constant Observation: Good Practice Guidelines for Healthcare Staff Working in Prisons*. The Stationery Office, London.

Doyle, M. (2000) Risk assessment and management. In: *Forensic Mental Health Nursing: Current Approaches* (eds C. Chaloner & M. Coffey), pp. 140–170. Blackwell Science, Oxford.

Kettles, A. & Paterson, K. (2007) Flexible observation: guidelines versus reality. *Journal of Psychiatric and Mental Health Nursing*, **14**(4), 373–381.

Kettles, A.M., Robinson, D. & Moody, E. (2003) A review of clinical risk and related assessments in forensic psychiatric units. *British Journal of Forensic Practice*, **5**(3), 3–12.

Morgan, S. & Wetherell, A. (2004) Assessing and managing risk. In: *The Art and Science of Mental Health Nursing: A Handbook of Principles and Practice* (eds I. Norman & I. Ryrie), pp. 208–240. Open University Press, Maidenhead.

Prins, H. (2002) Risk assessment: still a risky business. *British Journal of Forensic Practice*, **4**(1), 3–8.

Reed, V. & Woods, P. (2000) *The Behavioural Status Index: A Life Skills Assessment for Selecting and Monitoring Therapy in Mental Health Care*. Psychometric Press, Sheffield.

Ross, T., Woods, P., Reed, V., *et al.* (2008) Assessing living skills in forensic mental health care with the Behavioural Status Index: a European network study. *Psychotherapy Research*, **18**(3), 334–344.

Webster, C.D., Martin, M.L., Brink, J., Nicholls, T.L. & Middleton, C. (2004) *Manual for the Short Term Assessment of Risk and Treatability (START). Version 1.0, Consultation Edition*. St. Joseph's Healthcare, Hamilton, Ontario, and Forensic Psychiatric Services Commission, Port Coquitlam, British Columbia.

Woods, P. (2008) The forensic mental health nurse's role in risk assessment, measurement and management. In: *Forensic Nursing: Roles, Capabilities and Competencies* (National Forensic Nurses' Research and Development Group, eds A. Kettles, P. Woods & R. Byrt), Chapter 10. Quay Books, London.

Woods, P. & Kettles, A.M. (2007) Measurement of health and social functioning. In: *Forensic Mental Health Nursing: Forensic Aspects of Acute Care* (National Forensic Nurses' Research and Development Group, eds A.M. Kettles, P. Woods, R. Byrt, M. Addo, M. Coffey & M. Doyle), pp. 121–134. Quay Books, London.

Index

actuarial methods and clinical judgement in
    risk appraisal 22–3
actuarial tools 20–23
  mental disorder and criminality 21
  precision 20
  psychopathic tendencies 20
  risk assessment scales 58–60
  sex offending histories 20
  violence 20–23
actuarial/static variables 54–7
adjustment of risk scale 60–61
ADPIE (assessment, diagnosis, plan,
    intervention, evaluation) 167–77
age, and violence 117
alcohol 209
  assessment tools 217–19
  dual diagnosis, care pathway 213, 221–37
Alcohol Use Disorders Identification Test
    (AUDIT) 103
amphetamines 223
  ecstasy 205, 207
  methyl diethanol amine (MDEA) 205, 207
  methylenedioxy-amphetamine (MDA) 205,
    207
  methylenedioxymethamphetamine (MDMA)
    205, 207
anger and aggression 90–91
  risk assessment tools 20, 90–91
  threatening behaviour 124–5
  verbal aggression 124–5

Beck Depression Inventory 169
Beck Hopelessness Scale 96
behaviour 51–2
Behavioural Status Index (BEST-index) 87–90
benzodiazepines 210
blame culture 15–16
Brøset Violence Checklist (BVC) 67, 91–4

CAGE screening test 100
Canada, epidemiology of suicidal behaviour
    158
cannabis 202–3
cannabis, paranoid psychoses 223
Care Programme Approach (CPA) 13
  and risk management cycle 26

children
  healthy development 160–61
  (no) evidence of risk from drug-using
    parents 232
clinical/dynamic variables 54–7
clinician-based multidisciplinary risk
    assessment 19
cocaine 203–205, 223
cognitive behavioural therapy, treatment for
    substance misuse 227
contingency tables 51–2
correlation 50–51
crack cocaine 204–206
crisis resolution/home treatment teams 3
critical incident stress
  debriefing (CISD) 183–4
  management (CISM) 183–5
crystal meth 211
cue exposure, treatment for substance misuse
    225–6

dangerousness, vs risk 12–13, 52
DAST (Drug Abuse Screening Test) 100–101
day services, substance misuse 227
decision tree analysis, theory of risk 63–6
dependence, defined 201
depression 169–71
  Beck Depression Inventory 169
  CES-D 169
determinants of health (WHO) 156–60
  age 156–7
  culture 157–8
  gender 158
  genetics/biological factors 159–60
  self-neglect and vulnerability 158
  sexual orientation 159
  United Kingdom 158
detoxification, treatment of substance misuse
    226–7
drug abuse *see* substance misuse
Drug Abuse Screening Test (DAST)
    100–101
drug-induced psychosis 222–4
dual diagnosis 200, 212
  care pathway 221
  see also substance misuse

Dual Diagnosis Good Practice Guide (DH 2002) 212, 213

ecstasy (amphetamine) 205, 207
ethnicity, and violence, risk to others 117
event 51
evidence 53

forensic nursing
  current status 27
  overlaps with MHNs 27
forensic settings, risk assessment of substance misuse 235–7
future of risk assessment 247–9

gender, violence, risk to others 117
genetics/biological factors, suicidal behaviour 159–60
Gunn seven-step procedure, risk assessment 18–19

HCR-20 Assessing Risk for Violence 20, 22–4, 91, 92–3
heroin 202–203
  maintenance therapy 225

illegal or non-prescribed drugs *see* substance misuse; *named substances*
instruments for risk assessment 20–23, 244–6, 248–9
  actuarial methods and clinical judgement 22–3
  definitions 78–81
    equivalence 79
    internal consistency 79–81
    reliability 78
    stability 78–9
    validity and predictive validity 79–81
  education and training 248–9
  inappropriate use 81–4
    adapting content 82
    altering scores 82
    appropriate training or qualifications 82–3
    ignoring copyright 81–2
    instrument abuse 83–4
    stealing 82
  precision 20
  reliability and validity 78–81
  specific instruments for MHNs 84–104
    BEST and START 87–90, 244
    general and multiple risk 84–7
    historical, clinical and risk management (HCR-20) 91–3
    risk of substance abuse 97–103, 119–20
    risk to others 87–93, 109–42
    risk to self 93–7, 143–97
    spousal assault 90
    suicide scales 93, 96–9
  item weighting 59

ketamine 209
khat 210

lysergic acid diethylamide (LSD) 205, 208, 223

mental disorder and criminality, risk assessment tools 21
mental health issues
  substance misuse 214–19, 232–3
    assessment 217–19
mental health nurses (MHNs)
  clinical supervision and support 33
  communication 29–30
  concepts in everyday practices 9–10, 19
  dedicated care plans 34–6
  essential clinical skills 29
  leadership attitudes 36–7
  multidisciplinary teams (MDTs), concepts in everyday practices 9–10
  observational behaviours and recognition skills 30–31
  preceptorship 33–4
  risk assessment and management roles 12, 25–39
  teamwork within MDTs 31
    importance of 31
mental health services 4
methamphetamine 205, 207, 211
methyl diethanol amine (MDEA) 205, 207
methylenedioxy-amphetamine (MDA) 205, 207
methylenedioxy-methamphetamine (MDMA) 205, 207
Michigan Alcohol Screening Test (MAST) 102
mixing drugs 211
models, Risk Assessment Management and Audit System (RAMAS) model 18
multidisciplinary teams (MDTs), involvement of MHNs 31–3

numeracy 249–50

opiate withdrawal, symptoms 226–7
outreach services 3

policy, substance misuse 212–14
policy development 248
post traumatic stress disorder (PTSD) 184–5
preceptorship, MHNs 33–4
prediction of reoffending 54
prediction of violence 22, 113–14, 127
predictive validity 80–81
probability 50
psychiatric patients, violence, risk to others 110–13
psychiatric services, variability in practice 17
psychopathic tendencies, risk assessment tools 20
Psychopathy Checklist-Revised (PCL-R) 20
psychosis, drug-induced 222–4
psychotherapy 177–8
public safety, improvement in mental health services 16

Rampton Hospital, therapeutic security 28
Rapid Risk Assessment for Sexual Offence Recidivism (RRASOR) 20
Receiver Operating Characteristic (ROC) analysis 65, 67
relational security 53

reliability 61, 78–9
religion 153
research, risk assessment 249–50
residential rehabilitation, substance misuse 227
restriction, RMA assessors 62
risk
 vs dangerousness 12–13
 defined 11–12
 see also theory of risk
risk assessment 1–47, 16–19, 247–51
 approaches 250–51
 blame culture 15–16
 clinician's responsibility 16
 components of process 13–14
 concepts in everyday practice 9–10, 19
 consequences of failings 4–5
 crisis resolution/home treatment teams 3
 defined 2–3, 11
 future 247–9
 importance of information application by
  MHNs 19
 multidisciplinary risk assessment, base
  histories 19
 outreach services 3
 positive risk-taking 53
 predicting harmful behaviour 18
 process, inclusions 13–14
 public safety and improvement in mental
  health services 16
 recommendations and guidelines 14
 research 249–50
 service user costs 15
 standardising and simplifying risk language
  10–12
  change in language 11
  definitions 2–3, 11–12
  risk management defined 11–12
 tolerable risk 11–12
 validated risk assessment 14–15
 violence and mental disorder, procedure
  18–19
 see also instruments for risk assessment
Risk Assessment Management and Audit
 System (RAMAS) model 18
risk assessment tools 20–23, 244–6
 actuarial methods and clinical judgement
  22–3
 precision 20
 see also instruments for risk assessment
risk language, standardising and simplifying
 10–12
 change in language 11
 dangerousness vs risk 12–13
risk management 12–16, 68–71
 'best practice' 70
 defined 11–12
 forensic services 4
 integral role of MHNs 12
 positive risk management 71–3
 secondary measures 69
 service user costs 15
 training needs 23–5
Risk Management Authority (RMA) 61–3
risk management cycle 26, 68

risk scales, scores adjustment 60–61
risk to others *see* violence
risk variables, actuarial/static vs clinical/
 dynamic 54–7

safety
 centrality to good healthcare 1
 improvement in mental health services 16
security 53
self-harm
 epidemiology 149
 scales 96
 see also suicidal behaviour
self-neglect and vulnerability 158, 166–7
 ADPIE 167
Sex Offender Risk Appraisal Guide (SORAG)
 20
sexual orientation, suicidal behaviour 159
Short-Term Assessment of Risk and Treatability
 (START) 84–7, 244
SOAS-R (Staff Observation and Aggression
 Scale-Revised) 93, 95
social support networks 160–61
social theories, suicidal behaviour 152–3
socioeconomic status, suicidal behaviour 153
speed ball 211
spousal assault, specific instrument 90
Staff Observation and Aggression Scale-Revised
 (SOAS-R) 93, 95
START (Short-Term Assessment of Risk and
 Treatability) 84–7, 244
static variables 54–7
steroids, effects and risk factors 205, 208
stimulant drugs 203–11
substance misuse 97–103, 119–20, 126, 199–242
 alcohol 209
 assessment tools 217–19
 benzodiazepines 210
 care pathways 219–24
  drug-induced psychosis 222–4
  dual diagnosis 221
 class A, B and C drugs 202
 cycle of change 218
 dependence 201
 drug-induced psychosis 222–4
 engagement 224
 epidemiology 200
 harm minimisation 231–2
 illegal or non-prescribed drugs 201–11
  stimulant drugs 203–11
 ketamine 209
 khat 210
 lysergic acid diethylamide (LSD) 205, 208
 mental health issues 214–19, 232–3
  assessment 217–19
  maintaining mental health 237
  profile of service user group 214–17
 parental risk to children (lack of evidence)
  232
 policy 212–14
 publications 214
 risk assessment
  forensic settings 235–7
  and risk factors 232–3

substance misuse (*cont'd*)
  risk management
    forensic settings 235–7
    mental health settings 232–3
  scales 97–103
  steroids 205, 208
  treatment options 224–32
    cognitive behavioural therapy 227
    cue exposure 225–6
    detoxification 226–7
    prescribing 225
    relapse prevention 228–31
    residential rehabilitation 227
    risk reduction 231
    structured day services 227
  violence 119–20, 126
suicidal behaviour 143–97
  age 156–7
  assessment, diagnosis, plan, intervention,
    evaluation (ADPIE) 167–77
  child development 160–61
  clinical factors 155
  context of determinants of health (WHO)
    156–60
  continuum with harm by others 147
  culture 157–8
  definitions 145
  determinants of health (WHO) 156–60
  diagnosis, plan, intervention, evaluation
    (ADPIE) 167–77
  electroconvulsive therapy (ECT) 179
  epidemiology 149, 158
  etiology 149
    socio-cultural etiology 152–3
  gender 158
  genetics/biological factors 159–60
  legal considerations 182–3
  protective factors 154–6
  psychiatric illness and sociological issues
    150–51
  psychopharmacology 178–9
  psychotherapy 177–8
  religion 153
  risk and protective factors 154–6
    clinical factors 155
    precipitants and protective factors 156
  scales 96–7
  self-neglect and vulnerability 158, 166–7
  sexual orientation 159
  social support networks 160–61
  socioeconomic status 153
  stressors 172–3
  substance abuse treatment 179–81
  suicide by imitation 153–4
  terminology 146–7
  theories
    biologic 149–51
    psychological 151–2
    social 152–3
  vulnerability 164–6
  warning signs or invitations to help 162–4
    case study 164
suicide and trauma survivors 183–5
  critical incident stress debriefing (CISD) 183–4

critical incident stress management (CISM)
    183–5
  post traumatic stress disorder (PTSD) 184–5

teamwork *see* multidisciplinary teams (MDTs)
theory of risk 49–75
  actuarial risk assessment scales 58–60
  adjustment of risk scale scores 60–61
  Brøset Violence Checklist (BVC) 67
  causes of offending behaviour and inference
    58
  common terminology/definitions 49–54
  concept of risk management 68–71
    best practice points for effective risk
      management 70
  decision tree analysis 63–6
  defining terms 49–54
  validated scale scores, improvement of
    reliability 61
  variables 54–61
    dynamic risk variables 55–8
    stable and acute dynamic factors 57–8
    static (or actuarial) risk variables 54–6
therapeutic security, Rampton Hospital 28
THREAT assessment scale 85
threatening behaviour 124

validity 61, 79–80
  predictive 80–81
violence (risk) 109–42, 123–6
  and age 117
  assessing risk to others 133
  assessment 20–23, 114–16, 120–28
    considerations 128
    improving practice 132
    risk factors for violence 122, 133
    short- and long-term predictions 127
  exploitation of vulnerability 126
  management 21, 129–31
    improving practice 132
    insight and coping strategies 125–6
  mental state 125
  nurse–patient relationship 131
  offending behaviour 126
  patient-related variables 117–20
    diagnosis 118–19
    ethnicity 117
    gender and age 117
    prior history of violence 119
    substance abuse 119–20, 126
  potential victims 126
  prediction 22, 113–14, 127
  previous violence 124–5
  in psychiatric patients 110–13
  risk assessment tools 20–23
  risk factors for violence 122, 133
  stalking 124
  verbal aggression and threatening behaviour
    124
  see also suicidal behaviour
Violence Risk Appraisal Guide (VRAG) 20

WHO, determinants of health, suicidal
    behaviour 156–60